BASIC
Health, Hygiene and Safety

John L. Foster

Nelson

Acknowledgements

The author and publishers wish to thank the following who have kindly given permission for the use of copyright material:

Berkshire Family Practitioner Committee
Boots
British Red Cross Society
Controller of Her Majesty's Stationery Office
Elkington, Pat and Joan Ward ('Biology You Need')
Eva, Dave and Ron Oswald ('Health and Safety at Work')
Health Education Authority
Kinnersley, P. ('The Hazards of Work: How to Fight Them')
MENCAP
MIND
The Organisation of Chartered Physiotherapists in Private Practice
The Society of Chiropodists
Woman Magazine

The author and publishers wish to acknowledge, with thanks, the following photographic source:

Sally and Richard Greenhill

The publishers have made every effort to trace the copyright holders, but if they have inadvertently overlooked any, they will be pleased to make the necessary arrangements at the first opportunity.

Thomas Nelson and Sons Ltd
Nelson House Mayfield Road
Walton-on-Thames Surrey
KT12 5PL UK

Nelson Blackie
Wester Cleddens Road
Bishopbriggs
Glasgow G64 2NZ UK

Thomas Nelson Australia
102 Dodds Street
South Melbourne
Victoria 3205 Australia

Nelson Canada
1120 Birchmount Road
Scarborough Ontario
M1K 5G4 Canada

© J Foster 1988

First published by Macmillan Education Ltd 1988
ISBN 0-333-45133-3

This edition published by Thomas Nelson and Sons Ltd 1992

I(T)P Thomas Nelson is an International
       Thomson Publishing Company

I(T)P is used under licence

ISBN 0-17-438502-1
NPN 9 8 7 6 5 4

Printed in China

Contents

Introduction

This book forms part of a series designed for use by a wide range of students in school and further education, to provide practice in the development of core skills and knowledge in a variety of essential areas.

In particular, the series aims to ensure competence in core skills so that potential employees – school and college leavers – actually master the basic skills required by employers. Many of the skills included in the series are also needed in everyday life.

The approach taken is to present information in clear and carefully controlled steps and to provide numerous straightforward questions and tasks designed to test skills and explore the information presented.

The books are suitable for use not only with those pupils and students normally expected to take GCSE examinations, but also with those at all levels of ability, including students on pre-vocational courses such as CPVE and RSA Vocational Preparation. Each book is based upon the syllabus of the basic skills tests of the Associated Examining Board (Staff Hill House, Guildford, Surrey GU2 5XJ).

This book is targeted at the AEB Basic Health, Hygiene and Safety Test. It can be used in conjunction with the 'Basic Lifeskills' book, which also contains a number of sections giving basic information on health and safety matters.

The book is also designed to help those preparing for first aid tests by providing information about skills, techniques and procedures, and to give essential information to students and employees following a basic safety training programme.

Personal Health

In order to keep your body fit, you must take care of it by eating a healthy diet, exercising regularly and taking care with personal hygiene. You need also to be aware of the dangers to your health from smoking, alcohol and drug abuse.

A healthy diet

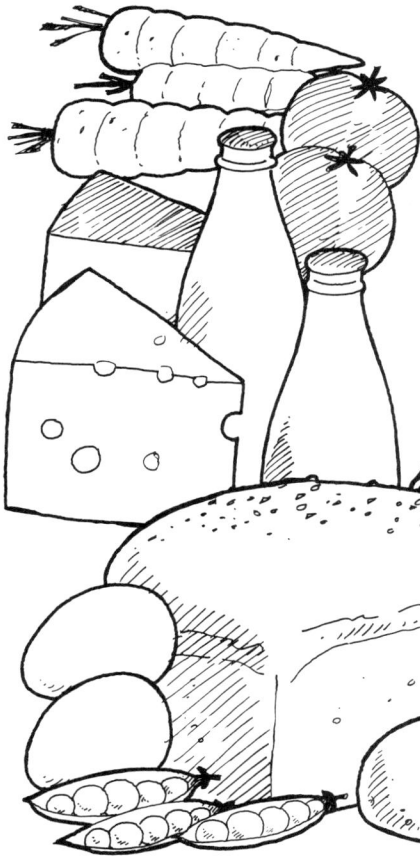

To keep healthy you need a balanced diet. Your body needs some body-building foods (proteins), some energy-giving foods (carbohydrates and fats) and some protective foods (vitamins and minerals). It also needs plenty of fibre which helps you to get rid of solid waste.

Your body needs the right amount of food. If you eat too much or too little, you are likely to get ill. In Britain, many people eat too much fat, sugar and salt. A healthy diet cuts down your chances of developing heart trouble and many other illnesses, such as constipation, bowel trouble and tooth decay.

A balanced, mixed diet contains the right foods to keep you healthy.

Fat

There are two types of fat: *saturated fats* and *unsaturated fats*. The unsaturated fats contain a group called *polyunsaturated fats*. Your body needs a small amount of polyunsaturated fats to help make and repair your body cells. Saturated fats are found in meat and dairy products, like milk, butter and cheese, in some vegetable oils, such as palm oil and coconut oil, and in cakes, biscuits, chocolates, cooking fats, hard margarines, sauces and puddings. Polyunsaturated fats are found in some vegetable oils, like sunflower, corn or soya oils, in some soft margarines, in nuts and in oily fish such as herring and trout.

Eating too much fat can make you overweight, because fat is full of calories. If you are overweight, you are more likely to get ill. Too much saturated fat increases your chances of getting heart disease. Saturated fat contains cholesterol which may damage your arteries.

Salt

Salt is present naturally in many foods. It is also added to a lot of manufactured foods during food processing.

You need some salt every day – about one gram. But on average we eat about ten grams of salt a day. Too much salt causes some people to get high blood pressure which is a cause of heart disease and strokes. At present, we can't tell which people are likely to get high blood pressure from eating too much salt.

Sugar

Many processed foods – biscuits and cakes, soft drinks, sweets and chocolates – contain sugar. Also, on average we buy a pound of sugar per person each week. Sugar is high in calories and provides you with energy. But it does not contain any protein, vitamins, minerals or fibre.

Eating too much sugar will make you overweight. If you don't use up the energy you get from eating sugary foods, then the energy will be stored as fat. Sugary foods also cause tooth decay. Sugar feeds the bacteria on your teeth. The bacteria then produce acid which causes tooth decay.

Fibre

Fibre is contained in the plant carbohydrates which we eat. They are found in the plants we grow to eat – cereals (wheat, corn, rice etc.), peas, beans, fruit and vegetables. Your body needs fibre because it helps you to get rid of solid waste and to keep your bowels healthy.

Good sources of fibre are wholemeal bread, breakfast cereals, vegetables, fruit and nuts. One advantage of eating foods that contain lots of fibre is that they fill you up without making you fat. Also, foods that are rich in fibre contain lots of vitamins and other nutrients. Too much fibre can rob the body of minerals.

Slimming diets

Many people are tempted to follow strict slimming diets which do not include a good balance of essential nutrients. In the long run, these are likely to do more harm than good. You should seek medical advice if you feel you have a serious weight problem.

Anorexia nervosa

This is a serious illness which mostly affects some teenage girls who feel they must lose weight in order to become attractive. Eventually they become obsessed with the idea that they must not eat. Such people need much love, reassurance and encouragement as well as medical treatment in order to become healthy again.

Tasks

1   Study the advice on healthy eating below. Work out the reason for each piece of advice.

Healthy eating tips
a) Whenever possible grill food rather than fry it.
b) When you are baking, use the wholemeal flour rather than plain flour.
c) Buy plain breakfast cereals instead of sugar-coated cereals.
d) Use skimmed or semi-skimmed milk rather than ordinary milk.
e) Eat more fish and chicken and less red meat.
f) Have a fresh fruit salad instead of tinned fruit.
g) Always fry chips in either corn oil, soya oil or sunflower oil.
h) Have a piece of fruit or some unsalted nuts as a snack instead of crisps or chocolate.
i) Eat home-made soups rather than tinned or packet soups.
j) Eat more beans, pulses and jacket potatoes and less fried foods.

2   Think up another five healthy eating tips to add to the list.

3   Here is what four people ate yesterday. Which of them do you think ate the most healthy

a) breakfast
b) lunch
c) dinner?

Overall, who do you think ate the healthiest diet?

	Nadia	**Les**	**Jo**	**Vicki**
Breakfast	bowl of muesli with milk, cup of coffee with milk	egg, two slices of bacon, piece of fried bread, cup of coffee with one sugar	glass of orange juice, bowl of cornflakes with skimmed milk, no sugar	two slices of toast and marmalade, cup of tea with two sugars
Lunch	hamburger in a bun with onions and dressing, large chips, small coke	steak and kidney pie, two packets of crisps, pint of beer	tin of soup, jacket potato with cheese filling, apple, glass of water	fish-paste sandwiches, yoghurt, carton of orange squash
Dinner	lamb chop, boiled potatoes, cauliflower, tinned peaches	fish fingers, mashed potatoes, peas, rhubarb crumble and cream	ham and salad, cheese and biscuits, orange	chicken curry with rice and poppadum

4   Write down everything you ate yesterday. Do you think you ate a healthy diet compared with the four people above?

5   What are your canteen meals like? Do they offer you a healthy diet? How much would it cost you to buy a healthy meal at your canteen? Would it cost you more? less? about the same? as a less healthy meal?

Exercise

Exercise strengthens your muscles and helps to keep them in good working order.

Exercise helps to keep your lungs in good condition. When you exercise, you breathe more quickly and deeply because you use up more energy and need more oxygen.

Exercise helps to keep your body supple. If you are supple, you are less likely to get injured.

Exercise builds up your strength and protects you from sprains and strains. If you are fit, you are less likely to hurt yourself pushing, pulling, lifting or carrying things.

Exercise helps you to control your weight. It uses up the calories in food which might otherwise be stored as fat.

Exercise helps to make your heart work more efficiently. It improves your circulation because it increases the rate at which the blood flows round the body. It builds up your stamina and helps to protect you against heart disease.

Exercise helps you to relax and keeps you mentally healthy as well as physically healthy.

To get fit and stay fit you need to take 20 or 30 minutes of exercise two or three times a week. Walking is a good form of regular exercise. You can help to keep yourself fit by using stairs rather than lifts when you are young and able-bodied!

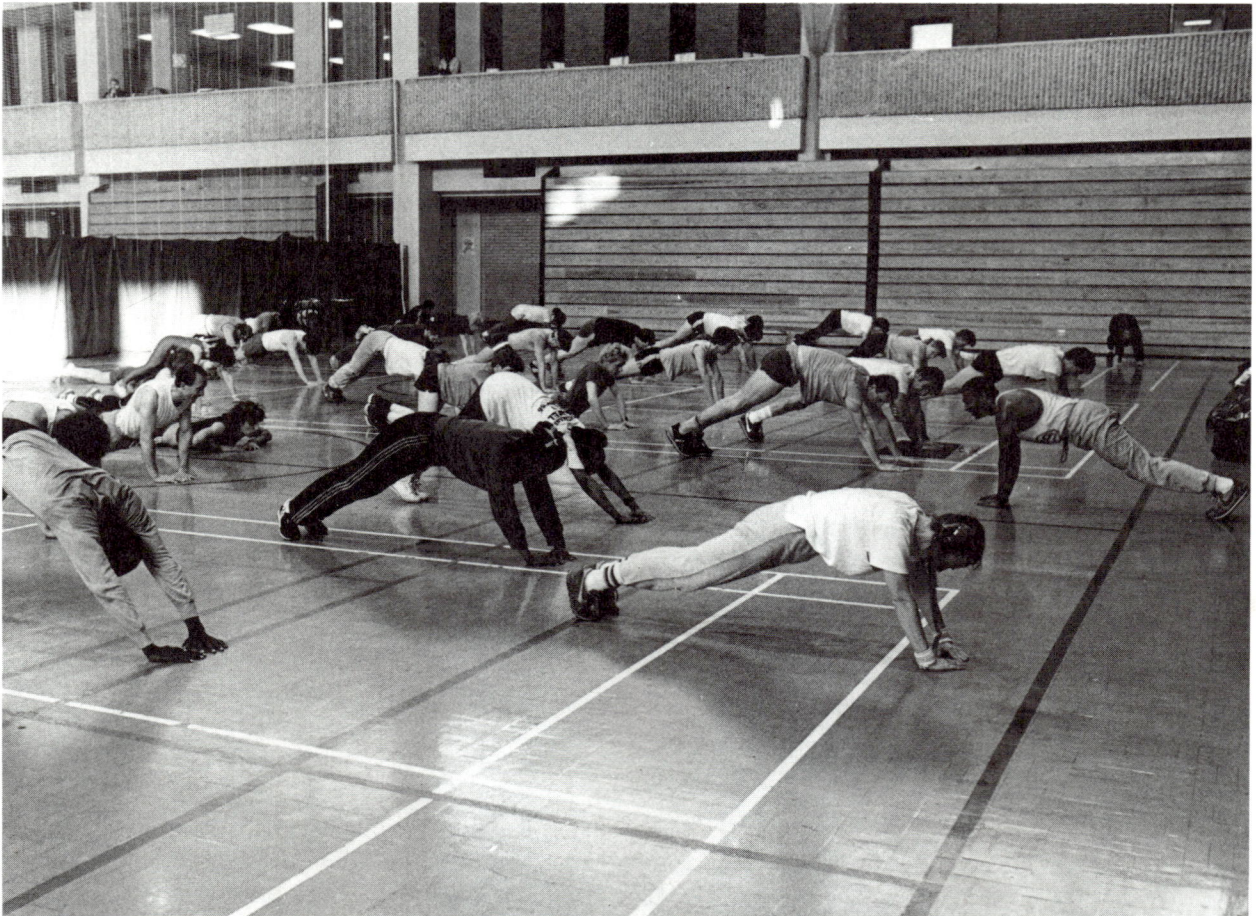

Regular exercise will help your body work more efficiently and will build up your strength.

1 What arguments would you use to convince someone who says exercise is a waste of time, that exercise is good for you?
2 Most people don't need a check-up before they start taking exercise. Explain why you should ask your doctor about the best form of exercise for you if you have
   a) high blood pressure or heart disease
   b) chest trouble like asthma or bronchitis
   c) back trouble or have had a slipped disc
   d) diabetes
   e) just had an operation or a serious illness.
3 If you have these symptoms, you should stop exercising: pain, dizziness, feeling unwell, unusual fatigue. Why?
4 A friend in your area wants to find an activity that will give her the exercise she needs. She wants an activity that she can do regularly outside working hours, near her home, that won't cost too much and that she can do all the year round. Suggest some activities for her to choose from.

Smoking

Cigarettes are harmful because tobacco smoke consists of about 300 different chemicals. When you smoke a cigarette, these substances enter your body through your mouth and lungs. The chemicals include nicotine, carbon monoxide, irritant substances and carcinogens.

- The effect of nicotine varies depending on the individual and the amount you inhale. *Nicotine* is a very powerful drug which passes into the bloodstream from the lungs. At first, it makes you more active. It causes a rise in blood pressure and makes your heart beat faster.
- *Carbon monoxide* is a deadly gas which affects the blood's ability to carry oxygen round your body. This is particularly important for people who have heart disorders or asthma. It is also harmful during pregnancy because it affects the supply of oxygen to the unborn baby.
- *Irritants* affect the cells in your air passage and lungs. In order to protect the cells, mucus is produced. Smokers cough in order to try to clear the irritants and the mucus.
- Tobacco tar contains a number of different substances. Some of these substances, known as *carcinogens*, have been shown to produce cancer in animals. When you inhale tobacco smoke, these substances pass into your lungs. They are present in smoke-filled air and can affect non-smokers who are in the same room as smokers.

Smoking-related diseases

The main smoking-related diseases are as follows:

Coronary heart disease Smoking is likely to damage your heart because the chemicals in cigarette smoke cause a rise in your blood pressure and an increase in your pulse rate. Coronary heart disease is one of the main causes of death in Britain. Cigarette smokers are about twice as likely to die of a heart attack as non-smokers.

Cancer Ninety per cent of the deaths from lung cancer are related to smoking. Smoking has also been linked with the growth of cancer in the mouth, larynx, pancreas and bladder.

Bronchitis The irritants in tobacco smoke produce mucus and cause smokers to cough. This makes the air tubes sore so that they swell and produce phlegm. A person who has bronchitis has difficulty in breathing and may start to wheeze. Seventy-five per cent of the deaths from bronchitis are caused by smoking.

Emphysema The small air sacs in the lungs may get damaged by coughing and bronchitis. As a result, the lungs can no longer function properly. A person with emphysema may be unable even to walk up a short flight of steps without getting very short of breath.

Smoking also contributes to a number of other diseases such as hardening of the blood vessels, blood clots and stomach ulcers.

How great are the risks from smoking?

- Not all smokers will suffer from one or more of the smoking-related diseases. But they are at much greater risk than non-smokers. For example, emphysema is rarely seen in non-smokers.
- Death from a smoking-related disease is more likely for a smoker than for a non-smoker. Ninety per cent of all deaths from lung cancer and chronic bronchitis are smokers. A study of civil servants and coronary heart disease showed that the death rate for cigarette smokers from CHD was 64–75% higher than for non-smokers.
- On average, a person who smokes 20 cigarettes a day shortens his or her life by 5 years and by about 5½ minutes for each cigarette smoked.

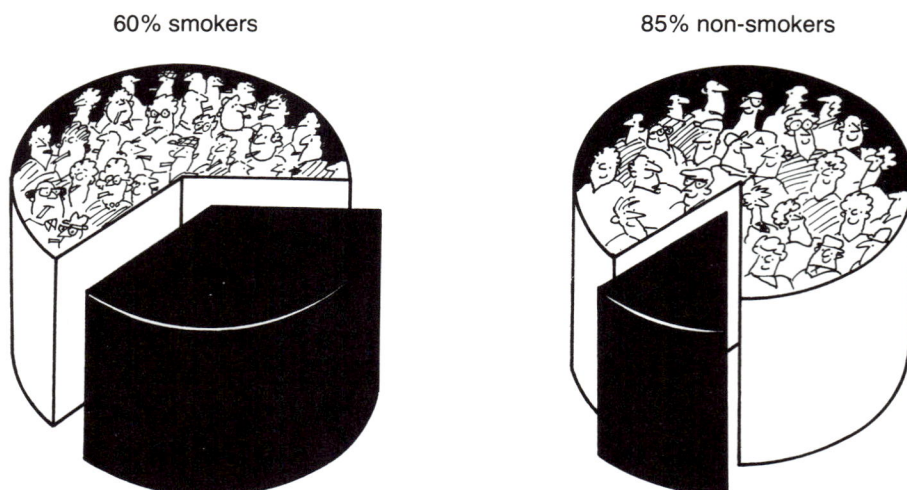

60% smokers   85% non-smokers

% of people who live beyond retirement age

- Forty per cent of heavy smokers (over 20 cigarettes a day) die before retirement age compared with only 15% of non-smokers. Most smokers will tell you about the fit, elderly and heavy smokers they know. But this doesn't mean they too will be one of the lucky ones.
- It is true that the effects of smoking are not always fatal. But most of the diseases related to smoking are either chronic or may lead to a diminished quality of life. For example, look at the lifestyle of a severely chronic bronchitic patient. He's on oxygen at home, is very ill each winter, needs help to cope with daily life and hardly ever leaves the house.
- One of the dangers of cigarette smoking is that it produces a dependence on and addiction to nicotine. Remember, it is estimated that two out of every three smokers either want to give up but can't bring themselves to try, or have tried and failed. Because of the addictive effect of the nicotine in cigarettes, the ex-smoker may suffer withdrawal symptoms at first, which may include depression, irritability, anxiety, tension, restlessness and lack of concentration. These symptoms may last for several weeks.

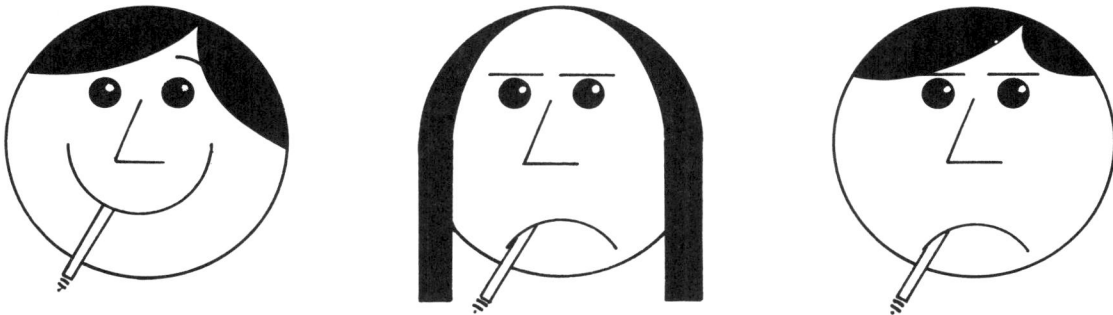

Two out of every three smokers want to give up.

Women and smoking

Women's health is affected by smoking. Over the last twenty years the pattern of disease in women smokers has been changing as it gradually becomes 'acceptable' for women to smoke. Between 1969 and 1978 lung cancer rates in women rose by more than 50% (only 8% in men). And they are still rising. The risk of circulatory and heart disease for a woman who smokes is especially high if she is over 35 and on the pill.

Smoking and pregnancy

If a woman smokes during pregnancy the carbon monoxide and nicotine from her cigarette are carried to the foetus via the placenta. This causes physiological changes in the unborn baby. Almost twice as many mothers who smoke have low birth-weight babies (under 5lb at birth) than non-smokers. And babies born to mothers who smoke are on average eight ounces lighter and have a one third greater perinatal mortality rate in the first month than babies born to mothers who don't smoke.

A mother-to-be should also be concerned about her own health. As well as the effects her smoking will have on her unborn child her own health is as much at risk as always.

Questions

1 Make up a test-yourself-quiz consisting of ten statements about smoking that are either True or False. Then give the quiz to someone in your group to do.
2 List the reasons why giving up smoking will improve your health.
3 What is 'passive smoking'? How may you be affected by cigarette smoking even if you do not smoke yourself?
4 In Belgium, smoking is now banned in public places. Do you think it should be banned in public places in Britain? Give your reasons.
5 Some people argue that cigarette smokers should have to pay for their own medical treatment, if they develop a smoking-related disease. What do you think?

Task

Find out about the work of ASH – Action on Smoking and Health, 5–11 Mortimer Street, London W1N 7RH.

Drinking

How much alcohol is there in different drinks? The alcohol content of different drinks varies. Beer contains about 5% alcohol, while in spirits and liqueurs the alcohol content is usually between 40% and 55%. One way of comparing the alcohol content of different drinks is to think of *standard drinks*, each of which contains the same amount of alcohol.

1 standard drink =

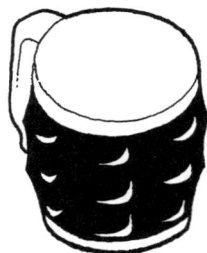

½ pint beer or ordinary lager

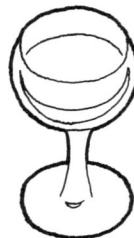

1 standard glass of wine

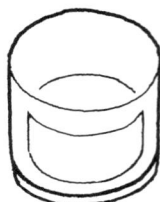

1 single measure of spirits (e.g. gin or whiskey)

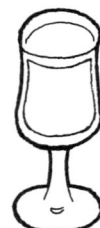

1 small glass of sherry

What happens when you drink alcohol?

When you drink alcohol, it goes into your stomach and is then absorbed into your bloodstream. It is carried to your brain and other parts of your body by your blood.

- How does alcohol affect you?
  It slows down your responses. Your brain does not work so quickly. That's why you are more likely to have an accident at work or on the roads after you have been drinking.
- How quickly does alcohol affect you?
  It usually takes about five or ten minutes for alcohol to start affecting you. It takes longer for the alcohol to enter your bloodstream if your stomach is full of food. So it is safer to drink alcohol after a meal than to begin to drink alcohol on an empty stomach.
- How quickly do the effects wear off?
  This will depend on how much alcohol you have been drinking. It takes about an hour for your body to get rid of the alcohol in one standard drink.
- How does your body get rid of alcohol?
  You get rid of some of the alcohol in your urine and your sweat, but most of it has to be burnt up by your liver. That's the reason why people who drink too much alcohol often damage their livers.
- Why do some people become alcoholics?
  Alcohol is a drug. If you regularly drink too much of it, your body starts to depend on it. An alcoholic is a person who cannot do without alcohol and has become addicted to it. An alcoholic can become both physically and mentally dependent on alcohol. The lives of an alcoholic's family can also be seriously affected by alcohol.
- Does alcohol affect men and women in the same way?
  No, women are more affected by alcohol than men. That's because a woman's body weight is made up of between 45% and 55% of water, but a man's body weight is made up of between 55% and 65% of water. So any alcohol a man drinks is more 'diluted' than it is in a woman. Also, it has been shown that alcohol is more likely to damage a woman's liver.
- Is it safe to drink when you are pregnant?
  Doctors think it is best not to drink when you are pregnant because if you drink alcohol, some of it will go to the baby. It is carried to your baby in the blood which carries food from you to the baby while the baby is in your womb.

Tasks

1 Work with a partner. Test each other by taking it in turns to read out the questions. See if your partner can answer the questions correctly without looking at the book.

2 Mark, Tony, Lee, Nadine, Gloria and Sue went to a pub. Mark went straight from work, so he had had no supper. He drank three pints of lager and ate two packets of crisps. The others had all had their suppers before going out. Tony had a pint of beer and two whiskies. Lee had three pints of lemonade shandy. Nadine had two grapefruit juices and a sherry. Gloria had three half-pints of lager. Sue had three glasses of wine.

a) Make a chart to show how many standard drinks each person had. Here's the start of such a chart.

Standard drinks					
Name	**Beer**	**Spirits**	**Wine**	**Sherry**	**Total**
Mark					

b) When they left the pub, which person do you think was most likely to be feeling drunk? Why?

3 There are licensing laws to control the sale of alcohol to young people and to control the hours when alcohol can be sold in pubs, off-licences and clubs. There are also laws about drinking and driving. Find out what these laws are. Do you think any of them should be changed?

4 Make up a True or False quiz consisting of ten questions about drinking. Here is the first question from such a quiz:
1 Alcohol speeds up your responses. True or False?
When you have made up your quiz, give it to a friend to do.

Drugs and drug abuse

A *drug* is a chemical substance which affects the way your mind or body works. Drugs are manufactured from chemicals obtained from plants, animals or minerals.

When you are ill, doctors often prescribe drugs to help you get better. Most drugs have benefitted mankind when prescribed by someone who knows how they work. Some drugs, called antibiotics (such as penicillin), help your body to kill the germs which cause diseases. Other drugs, called analgesics (such as aspirin), act as painkillers. Another group of drugs, called tranquillisers (such as Valium), act to calm you down if you are anxious or under stress.

All drugs, including medicines, nicotine and alcohol, can be harmful if used irresponsibly. There are drugs which you can buy at the chemists which can become habit-forming, such as laxatives and cough mixtures. When legally controlled drugs are used without a doctor's prescription, then they are *illegal*. This group of illegal drugs includes barbiturates, amphetamines, LSD, cannabis, heroin and cocaine.

How do drugs work?

You can take a drug by swallowing, inhaling or injecting it. A drug which is swallowed dissolves in your stomach, then passes into your bloodstream. A drug which is inhaled passes into your bloodstream from your lungs. A drug which is injected goes straight into your blood.

The drug is carried to your brain by your blood. Your brain is constantly receiving and sending messages to and from the other parts of your body along your nerves. When a drug reaches your brain, the brain is affected and alters the messages it is sending out. Some drugs can cause permanent damage to the brain cells.

Different drugs affect the brain in different ways.
Stimulants speed up the way your brain works; they include cocaine, amphetamines.
Depressants slow down the way your brain works; they include barbiturates.
Hallucinogens affect your brain so that you see things differently. They are called hallucinogens because they cause visions or hallucinations, for example LSD (acid). Some solvents (e.g. glue, cleaning fluids) produce effects similar to alcohol or anaesthetics when their vapours are inhaled.

How a drug affects you varies from person to person because we each have our own individual body chemistry. The effects also depend on other factors such as your body weight, your general health, the amount you take, the mood you are in and the situation in which the drug is taken.

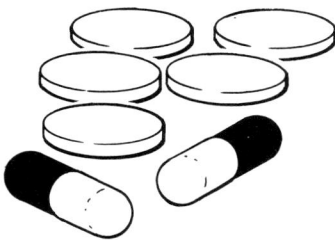
amphetamines

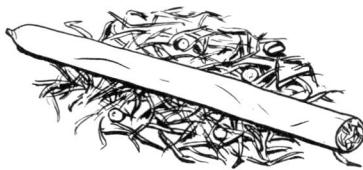
cannabis

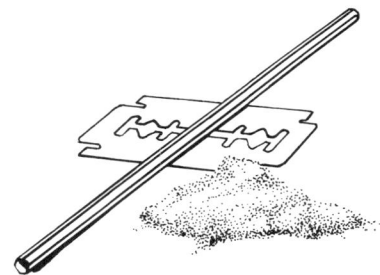
cocaine

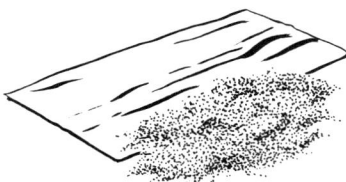
heroin

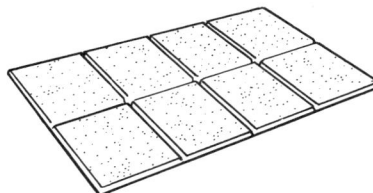
LSD

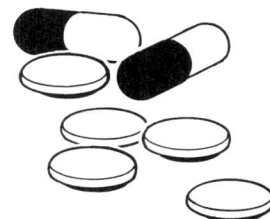
tranquillisers

When these drugs are misused, they can cause many problems.

Drug abuse

Some people start taking drugs without being prescribed them by a doctor. If they go on taking drugs regularly, they may become ill or dependent on drugs. That's why it is an offence to possess or supply drugs like heroin and cocaine without a doctor's authorisation.

You can become dependent on drugs in two ways. If you get so used to taking drugs that you feel you can't cope without them, you are *psychologically dependent* on drugs. If your body gets so used to drugs that you feel physically ill without them, then you are *physically dependent* on drugs.

A person who tries to stop taking a drug such as heroin will suffer from withdrawal symptoms, which make him or her feel physically ill. That's what makes it so hard for people to give up taking heroin.

Cannabis is called a 'gateway' drug. This is because people who start on cannabis often find that they want a stronger drug, such as heroin.

People who inject drugs are more at risk than other drug users, because they sometimes share needles and syringes. Sharing dirty needles and syringes can pass on infections from one person's blood into another person's bloodstream. Addicts who share needles and syringes run the risk of catching AIDS.

Drug addicts who want to stop taking drugs can be given treatment for their addiction. A lot of people have been rehabilitated. However, others manage to give up drugs for a while, then find they cannot resist the temptation to start taking drugs again.

Jason's story

Jason is 18. He is a drug addict. A year ago he was on a YTS course, living happily at home and had a steady girlfriend.

Now he's unemployed, in trouble with the police for shoplifting to pay for his habit and his girlfriend has told him she doesn't want to have anything more to do with him. It all started a year ago when he was at a party and he was offered a cannabis joint.

'My mind wasn't straight at the time and they said it would calm me down,' he said.

After three months, he tried 'speed' (amphetamine sulphate), then cocaine, then finally heroin.

'I was at a party and we were showing off the first time I took heroin. I just wanted to look cool. I was really happy and talkative after I'd taken heroin but I felt terrible when I came down.

I haven't been on heroin very long, but it's screwing up my life. I'm determined to try and give it up, so I'm going to this treatment centre but I'm scared I won't be able to stop using heroin.'

Tasks

1 a) State three medical uses of drugs.
  b) Name three drugs which cannot be used without a prescription and say why.
  c) Why do injected drugs affect you faster than drugs you swallow or inhale?
  d) Explain the difference between stimulants, depressants and hallucinogens.
  e) Why does the same drug affect different people in different ways?
2 a) List the reasons why a person might start taking drugs.
  b) What's the difference between psychological dependence and physical dependence?
  c) What do you learn about how drug-taking affects a person's life from reading Jason's story?
3 If you found that your 15-year-old sister or brother was taking drugs, what would you do? List all the factors you would consider in making your decision.
4 How serious a problem is drug abuse? Should the laws on drugs and drug abuse be changed? Should drug offenders be treated more harshly? Find out more information about drug abuse and prepare either a short talk or a short article stating your views.

Personal hygiene – Your feet

Each foot consists of 26 small, delicate bones with many ligaments and muscles. Your feet are specially designed to support the weight of your body. They are subject to more pressure and to more injury than any other parts of your body.

Basic rules of foot care

- All feet should be measured for shoes when you are standing. When buying shoes, check that you can wiggle your toes. If you cannot do so, the shoes are too tight.
- Avoid tight-fitting hosiery. A baby's feet can be pulled out of shape by wearing all-in-one stretch suits that are too small.
- Keep your feet clean and use a foot powder.
- Always wash and dry carefully between the toes.
- Trim your toenails longer than the top of your toe.
- Do not cut your own corns, callouses or ingrowing toenails. Either consult your doctor or see a state registered chiropodist.
- Avoid so-called corn 'cures', harsh medications or chemical compounds.
- Seek treatment promptly for burns, cuts, breaks in the skin or other unusual changes.

Some common foot ailments

- *Corns* are small areas of hardened skin on the tops of toes, which press inwards and can be very painful. Corns are caused by friction and pressure, usually from badly-fitting shoes.

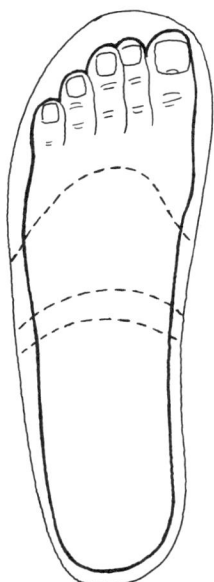

Shoes should fit comfortably to allow free movement of toes. If shoes are too tight, corns and bunions can result.

17

- *Callouses* are areas of hardened skin, usually on the sides or the soles of the foot, which can make walking painful. They are also caused by pressure from shoes.
- *Verrucae* are a type of wart that occurs on the sole of the foot. They are contagious and children often pick up the infection in swimming-baths. They tend to spread if they are untreated.
- *Bunions* are painful swellings of the big toe joint. They are caused by badly-fitting shoes, often when a young person's foot is pushed out of shape by wearing shoes with pointed toes.
- *Athletes's foot* is a skin disease which results in patches of white flaking skin between the toes and can cause itching and burning. It is caused by a fungus, which thrives on warm, moist skin.
- *Ingrowing toenails* are usually caused by incorrect trimming. When the nail grows, it grows into the flesh of the toe causing painful swelling.

Questions

1 Why are fashion-shoes often bad for your feet?
2 Why should you check a child's shoe size regularly every 8–10 weeks?
3 Why are parents encouraged to let children go barefoot whenever it is safe?
4 What usually causes ingrowing toenails?
5 What is the difference between a corn and a callous?
6 How are bunions caused?
7 What should you do if you get a verruca?
8 What are the symptoms of athlete's foot? How can you protect yourself against athlete's foot?
9 Why should you avoid handing down shoes from child to child or buying secondhand shoes?
10 Suggest three tips for how to keep your feet healthy.

Personal hygiene – Your teeth

The number of people with dental problems is declining. But about 80% of the people in Britain still suffer from some tooth decay and over 90% of us suffer from gum disease.

What causes tooth decay?

Tooth decay (dental caries) is caused when sugar reacts with plaque. Plaque is a sticky colourless film, consisting of food debris and saliva, which forms on your teeth. Bacteria grow in the plaque. These bacteria change sugar into acids. The acids then attack the enamel which forms the outer layer of your tooth. Tiny holes are made and if they are not treated the acids will eat through into the layers of dentine and pulp inside the teeth.

You can protect yourself against tooth decay.

- Clean your teeth regularly and properly.

- Change your diet so that you do not eat so many foods which contain sugar.
- Use a toothpaste with fluoride in it.
- Eat foods such as milk, cheese and eggs, which contain a lot of calcium.

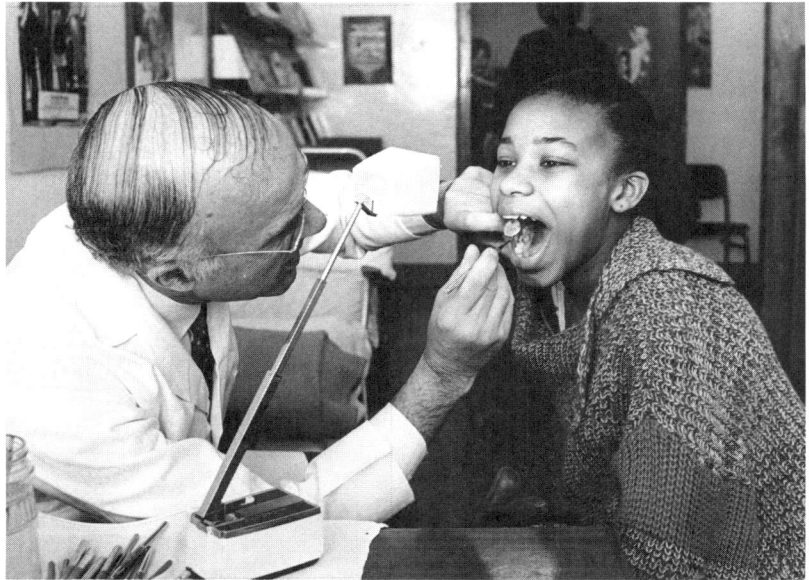

Careful brushing and regular dental check-ups help protect your teeth.

What causes gum disease?

You are more likely to lose teeth through gum disorders than through tooth decay. Gum disease often starts at about the age of 25. It is not caused by age but by lack of proper cleaning. If the plaque that collects around and under the gum margin is not cleaned away, the gums will swell. This may cause bleeding when you brush your teeth. Such bleeding is often the first sign of gum disease.

Over a period of time, the disease destroys the fibrous connections between the gum and the tooth. The bone structure that supports the tooth is exposed to attack. This can lead to a loosening of the tooth and loss of teeth in middle age.

toothache   **gum disease**

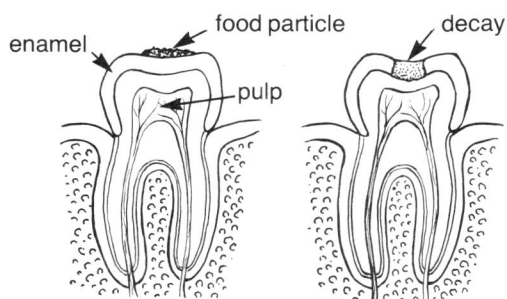
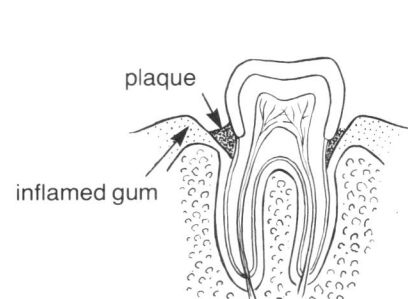

Toothache and gum disease are caused by a build-up of plaque.

Questions

1 What is dental plaque? Explain how plaque can cause
   a) tooth decay
   b) gum disorders.
2 What are the arguments for and against adding fluoride to drinking water? Does the drinking water in your area contain fluoride?

Tasks

1 Prepare a dental care factsheet to distribute to pupils at your local junior or middle school.
2 Prepare similar factsheets on hair care, skin care and eye care.

Mental health

Many people get confused about the difference between mental illness and mental handicap. These extracts from a leaflet produced by the National Association for Mental Health explain the difference.

In fact, mental illness and mental handicap are totally different. To understand how different they are, it helps to compare them, fact for fact.

Illness	*Handicap*
People *become* mentally *ill* when they can no longer cope with the stresses and problems in their lives.	People *are* mentally handicapped because they have a brain which will not develop as quickly or function as well as other people's.
Mental illness is often a temporary condition. It can be treated successfully, although the possibility of a relapse can never be ruled out.	Mental handicap is permanent, but people *can* be helped to overcome their disabilities with the right kind of education and support from the community in which they live.
One person in six will be affected by mental illness at some point in their life.	One person in every hundred is born mentally handicapped.
Although some people are more *likely* to become mentally ill than others, it is impossible to predict who will be affected.	Although some women run a slighty higher risk of giving birth to a handicapped baby, it is impossible to pinpoint accurately the one couple in every hundred who will have a mentally handicapped child.
There are any number of reasons why people become mentally ill. Unemployment, poor housing conditions, family difficulties, pressures at work or school, isolation and loneliness can all result in the kind of stress that some people are unable to deal with. There can be biochemical causes too – this is true in the case of schizophrenia – and some personality types are more likely to become mentally ill than others. People who have had an unstable family life are also more at risk as they grow up. For most people it's impossible to say that any one factor caused the mental illness: usually it's a combination of factors working together.	People who are mentally handicapped are usually born with this disability. Sometimes, the baby's brain is damaged during a difficult birth; sometimes there are problems during pregnancy – perhaps hormone deficiencies or German measles – which result in a woman giving birth to a mentally handicapped child. Down's Syndrome, the most common form of mental handicap, is caused by a genetic factor – the presence of an extra chromosome. Children who are born without any disabilities can become mentally handicapped through injury in an accident or through the after-effects of a vaccination or a disease such as meningitis.

Illness	Handicap
Mental illness can be treated in a number of ways. *Psychotropic* (mood altering) drugs can be used to give people the energy and confidence to deal with some of their problems. *Electro-convulsive therapy* (ECT) is a very controversial treatment, but it is effective in helping people suffering from severe depression. Talking treatments help people to gain an insight into the cause of their difficulties, and to come to terms with the problems. A combination of some or all of these treatments can and does restore many people to their usual way of life.	Because mental handicap isn't an illness or a medical problem, you can't talk in terms of treatments or cures. However, there is a lot that can be done to help people who are mentally handicapped. What they need most is education in the practical skills of everyday living, and social support to help them live as independently as their abilities will allow.
People who are mentally ill can't become mentally handicapped, unless their brains are seriously injured in an accident.	People who are mentally handicapped can also become mentally ill; they are as likely to be affected as anyone else. When this happens they can be treated medically, in the same way as other people who are mentally ill.

Questions

Study the information on these pages, then work out whether the following statements are True or False.

1. Mental illness is like physical illness. You can develop it at any point in your life.
2. A mentally handicapped person is not born with a mental handicap, but develops it during the first five years of life.
3. Mental illness can be cured.
4. A mental handicap lasts for life. People with mental handicaps can be educated and supported but cannot be cured.
5. Mental illness is very common.
6. The chances of a person having a mentally handicapped child are very slight.
7. It is possible to predict which people are likely to develop mental illness.
8. You cannot predict which couples are likely to have a mentally handicapped baby.
9. There is usually more than one cause of mental illness.
10. Mental handicap can be caused either by a difficult birth or by problems during pregnancy.
11. If you become mentally ill, you can develop a mental handicap.
12. People who are mentally handicapped can become mentally ill just like anyone else.

Task

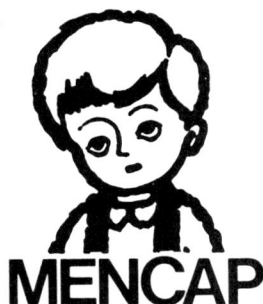

A *phobia* is an irrational and uncontrollable fear. Find out what agoraphobia is. How can people with agoraphobia be helped? (Information can be obtained from MIND, National Association for Mental Health, 22 Harley Street, London W1N 2ED and The Phobics Society, 4 Cheltenham Road, Chorlton-cum-Hardy, Manchester 21.)

MENCAP

MENCAP is a society which aims to increase public awareness and understanding of the problems of people with a mental handicap.

The National Health Service

When you are ill you are entitled to medical attention provided by the National Health Service.

Finding a doctor

Everyone has a right to be on a doctor's list of patients. If you are 16, you can choose your own doctor. Children under 16 have to go to a doctor chosen for them by a parent or a guardian. If you can't find a doctor to accept you, your local Family Practitioner Committee will find one for you.

If you are not satisfied with your doctor, you can apply to join another doctor's list. You don't have to say why you want to change doctors.

Medical cards

Everyone is issued with a medical card at birth. It has your NHS number on it.

NATIONAL HEALTH SERVICE	
MEDICAL CARD ISSUED BY THE Berkshire Family Practitioner Committee Great Western House, Station Road, Reading RG1 1LU	

Please notify your Doctor and the Family Practitioner Committee of change of name or address. Please quote your name and NHS Number on all correspondence.

Name

Address

NHS Number	Date of Birth
Dr.	Date issued
Code	FPC Cipher

NHS Number	Date of Birth
Dr.	Date accepted

Part A To be completed if you want to change your doctor.
Application to be placed on the list of Dr. .... Date ....

`*`Drugs

Signature of applicant ‡ ....
Address of Applicant ....
....

⁺ Rural Practice

Signature of accepting Doctor ....
Drs. Code No. .... Date ....

Part B

I agree to this transfer. Signature of consenting Doctor ....
Drs. Code No. .... Date ....

‡ A person signing for the applicant should state relationship
`*`If Doctor is to supply drugs he should enter D in space marked `*`
⁺ If Doctor claims a rural practice payment he should enter in the space marked ⁺ the distance from his main surgery to the patient's residence and should inform the Family Practitioner Committee if he wishes to claim for units in addition to those for ordinary distance

FP4 (COMP)

This is the more recent type of NHS card which is being issued to patients. It is linked to computerisation.

Medical treatment

You can get medical treatment by going to your doctor's surgery. To get hospital treatment you must be sent to the hospital by a doctor. However, if you have an accident, you can get emergency treatment at a hospital casualty department. Also, you don't need a doctor's letter in order to go to a special clinic for the treatment of VD and sexually transmitted diseases.

If you are 16, you can give or refuse your consent to any medical or surgical care, but most hospitals require a parent's permission to perform operations on anyone under 18.

Family planning clinics

You can get advice on contraception either from your family doctor or your nearest family planning clinic. There are NHS family planning clinics all over the country. You can get the address and times of your nearest clinic from your health centre, a midwife, hospital, health visitor or the telephone directory (under family planning). You do not need a doctor's letter before you go to a family planning clinic.

Charges

There is no charge for being seen by your doctor or for hospital treatment, but there is a charge for each item on a prescription. If you have to use drugs regularly, you can get a four-monthly or a yearly 'season ticket' from your Family Practitioner Committee.

Certain groups of people get free prescriptions: children under 16, pregnant women, people over retirement age, people claiming income support. If you have a road accident, doctors and hospitals can charge you for the emergency treatment they give you. The fees have to be paid either by the drivers of the vehicles involved or their insurance companies.

Dental treatment

You can obtain dental treatment either privately or under the National Health Service. Only some National Health Service treatment is free. If you are over 16 you have to pay for part of the cost of the treatment unless you belong to a group of people (such as pregnant women) who qualify for free treatment.

You can get a list of dentists who accept people for National Health Service treatment from the following places: a main post office, your local library, the Citizens Advice Bureau, your local Family Practitioner Committee or Community Health Council.

Eye care

New legislation has been proposed on the free eye-test, and there is likely to be a charge in the future. If you are over 16 and need glasses, you will have to pay the full cost of the lenses and frames, unless you belong to a group (such as people on income support) who qualify for a voucher towards part of the cost or are in full-time education. Contact lenses are not available under the National Health Service.

Tasks

1 Prepare a factsheet about the National Health Service services available in your area. Include the following:
   - Names, addresses and telephone numbers of doctors and their surgeries and details of surgery hours
   - Details of the local health centre, family planning clinic and ante-natal clinic
   - Address of the nearest hospital with a casualty department
   - Addresses and telephone numbers of dental surgeries and opticians
   - Names of chemists and details of how to find their duty rota
   - Addresses and telephone numbers of your local Family Practitioner Committee and Community Health Council.
   Sources of information you could use are: libraries, telephone directories, newspapers, Citizens Advice Bureau.

2 a) If you are going abroad, other than to an EEC country, it is a good idea to take out medical insurance. Why?
   b) If you are going to an EEC country, you should obtain a form E111. Why? Where can you obtain it?

3 If you were in charge of the health service in your area, what would your priorities be? Put 1 against your first choice, 2 against your second choice and so on down the list. Compare your order of priorities with other people's and discuss together how you decided your priorities.
   a) Closing a local maternity home in order to fund a new high technology maternity wing in the hospital
   b) Continuing to fund a unit working on 'test-tube' babies
   c) Running an advertising campaign to persuade local people to take more exercise
   d) Developing a screening programme for breast cancer
   e) Funding a unit to carry out heart transplants
   f) Supporting research into drugs to treat cancer
   g) Setting up local 'stop smoking' clinics
   h) Providing enough kidney machines to meet all known local needs
   i) Renovating the geriatric ward in the hospital
   j) Opening a community hostel for people with mental handicap

Health and Hygiene in the Community

Health and hygiene in the community are also important for your well-being. Diseases are spread from one group of people to another and it is necessary to fight the spread of disease.

Diseases

An *infectious disease* is a disease you can pass on to another person. The germs which cause infectious diseases are either bacteria, viruses or fungi. Germs can enter your body through your body openings (nose, mouth, sex organs, back passage), your skin or any wounds such as cuts, sores or insect-bites.

How infectious diseases are spread

By droplets Tiny droplets containing germs are coughed, sneezed or breathed out by an infected person. You breathe them in and become infected. Diseases spread in this way include colds, flu, measles and mumps.

By contact Some diseases are spread by contact. You touch something that is infected and catch the disease yourself. Diseases spread by contact are known as contagious diseases. Examples of contagious diseases are venereal diseases and many skin diseases, such as athlete's foot.

In water Germs that can live in water cause many diseases including typhoid, cholera and dysentry, as well as skin and eye infections, some of which can cause blindness. Drinking dirty water is one of the chief ways that infectious diseases are caught in many parts of the world.

In food Germs can develop on food that is kept for too long, not stored properly or cooked properly. Such germs, such as salmonella, will give you food-poisoning.

By insects Flies and other insects carry germs which they may deposit if they land on your food. Some insects infect you when they bite you. For example, you may catch malaria if you are bitten by a certain type of mosquito.

By animals Rats and mice spread germs. If your home is infested, you should call in the pest control officer. You can also catch diseases from your pets if you do not look after their health and handle them carefully.

Inherited diseases

An inherited disease is one that is passed on to you by your parents. Examples of inherited diseases are the blood conditions haemophilia and sickle cell diseases.

Haemophilia People with haemophilia do not have the substance in their blood which makes blood clot. So even a small cut can be very dangerous and lead to a blood transfusion.

Sickle cell disease The most common form of sickle cell disease is sickle cell anaemia. In Britain, one in ten black people carry the disease and 5000 people suffer from it. It affects red blood cells making them crescent or sickle shaped instead of round. These sickle cells clump together (sickling) and sometimes get stuck in the small blood vessels. This prevents the normal blood flow and is very painful.

People with sickle cell anaemia are likely to get bouts of anaemia, pain, jaundice or infections. These are known as *crises*. The frequency of crises varies from person to person. Some people have them only once every few years, others have them more often. As yet, there is no known cure, but research is going on to try to find a drug to prevent sickling.

Tasks

1 What is the difference between an infectious disease, a contagious disease and an inherited disease? Give an example of each type.
2 List the different ways that infectious diseases are spread.
3 List common infectious diseases and their symptoms. Which ones have you had? Carry out a survey to find out what the most common infectious diseases are these days.
4 Drains, dustbins, toilets and dirty washing are all potential sources of infection. Why? What hygiene precautions can you take to prevent infection in the home?
5 In the past, children with infectious diseases were often kept in quarantine. What is quarantine? Why is it not often observed nowadays?
6 List some hygiene rules for pet care to help to protect you from catching diseases from your pet.

Preventing infectious diseases

Many infectious diseases are now far less common than they used to be, because of higher standards of public health and the development of preventative medicine.

How your body fights disease

If the germs which cause an infectious disease enter your body, the white cells in your blood try to destroy them. The white cells produce special chemicals called *antibodies* which destroy germs or make them harmless.

The antibodies only fight the germs which cause one particular disease. Once they have been produced, they stay in your blood and protect you from getting that particular disease again. The antibodies are said to have made you immune from that disease.

Immunisation

Today, you can be given substances called vaccines which will protect you from catching certain infectious diseases. Some vaccines contain antibodies. Others work by making your body produce the antibodies it needs.

The chart below shows a typical vaccination programme.

Age		Protect against
3 months	1	diphtheria, tetanus, whooping cough*
	2	polio†
4 months	1	diphtheria, tetanus, whooping cough
	2	polio
5 months	1	diphtheria, tetanus, whooping cough
	2	polio
12 months		measles
18 months	1	diphtheria, tetanus, first booster whooping cough
	2	polio
4½–5 years	1	diptheria, tetanus second booster
	2	polio
11–13 years		(girls only) German measles
10–14 years		BCG vaccination against TB
15–19 years	1	tetanus
	2	polio

* these three are usually given in a single injection
† this is given in a teaspoon or, to older children, on a lump of sugar

There is no need for anyone to die of any of these diseases in the UK today but only people who have been immunised are protected against them.

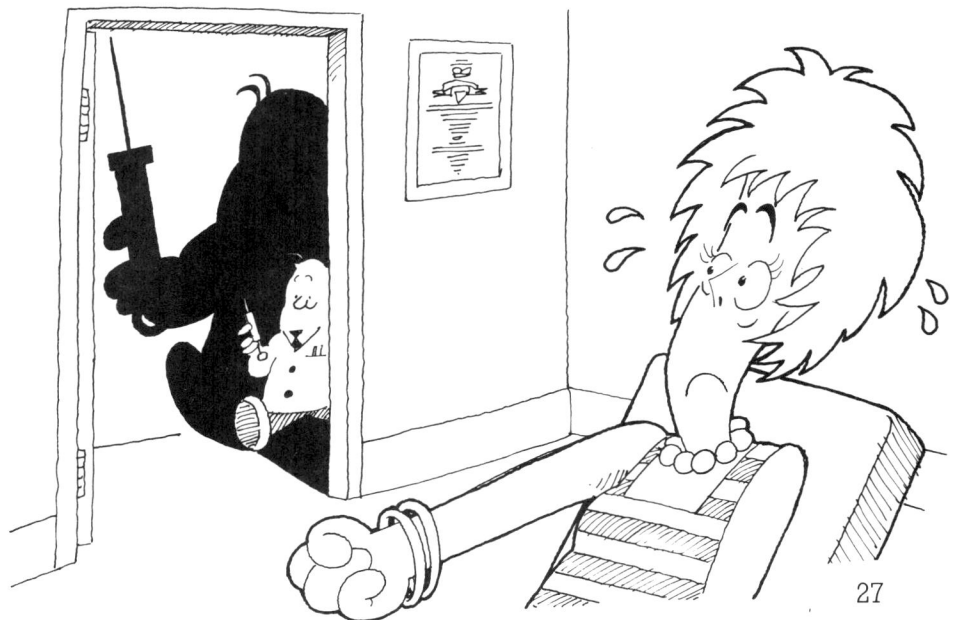

German measles

This is a very infectious disease. Its symptoms are a mild pink rash on your chest and a light fever. It usually lasts only a few days and you may not even realise you have it.

But if you catch German measles when you are pregnant, it can seriously damage your unborn baby. The baby may be born handicapped, with serious damage to its sight, hearing, brain or heart.

It is unusual to catch German measles twice, but its symptoms can easily be confused with those of other similar diseases. So it is hard to know for certain whether or not you have had it. That's the reason why doctors advise all girls between 10 and 14 to have an injection to immunise them against German measles.

Task

Use the information on diseases to solve the crossword below.

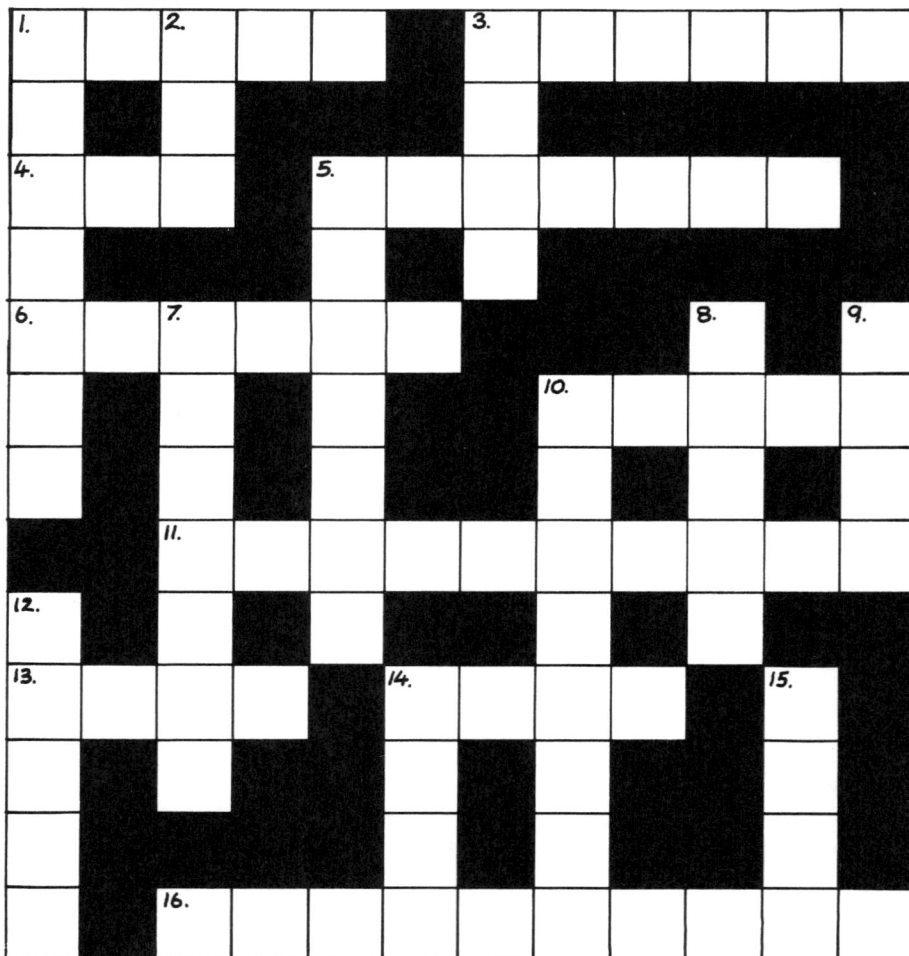

Clues across

1 A type of germ that causes diseases such as colds, flu, chicken pox and mumps (5)
2 People who suffer from sickle cell disease get these from time to time (6)
4 Even a small one of these can be dangerous for a haemophiliac (3)
5 You could catch this from drinking dirty water (7)
6 Protected against a disease (6)
10 A disease causing paralysis against which you can be vaccinated (5)
11 One in ten black people in Britain carry this disease (6,4)
13 Vital organs which can sometimes be damaged by germs carried in dirty water (4)
14 Eat food that has been kept too .... and you may get salmonella (4)
16 You need a series of these to vaccinate you against diphtheria, tetanus and whooping cough (10)

Clues down

1 If you are given this it will make you immune to a disease (7)
2 Animal that spreads germs (3)
3 A haemophiliac's blood cannot do this (4)
5 The way you catch a contagious disease (7)
7 You can be vaccinated against this at 12 months (7)
8 Insects which often deposit germs when they land on food or drink (5)
9 Do this to water to kill any germs in it (4)
10 German measles is not a harmless disease if you are in this condition (8)
12 Bacteria and viruses (5)
14 Many people do this longer because vaccination protects them against diseases that used to be common (4)
15 This protects your body but germs may enter through it if it is damaged (4)

Sexually transmitted diseases

Venereal diseases – commonly known as VD – are caught by having intimate sexual contact with an infected person. The three most common types of VD are non-specific urethritis (NSU), gonorrhoea and syphilis.

What are the symptoms of NSU?

In a man the tube which runs from the bladder to the tip of the penis is called the urethra. NSU causes an inflammation of the urethra known as urethritis. A man suffering from NSU has a discharge from the end of his penis and will feel discomfort passing water. A woman with NSU often has no symptoms.

What are the symptoms of gonorrhoea?

The symptoms of gonorrhoea appear in a man between about two and ten days after he becomes infected. He will feel pain when passing water and has a yellowish discharge leaking from his penis. In a woman, the germs cause inflammation of the opening of the womb, but this is not usually painful. Also, the discharge that is produced may not be noticed. Sometimes, the germs cause inflammation of the passage from the bladder and the woman may feel pain when passing water. But in the early stages there are often no obvious symptoms in a woman who has gonorrhoea.

However, if gonorrhoea is not treated, the germs will spread and cause inflammation to other parts of the body in both men and women. It can cause general ill-health, swollen joints and permanent damage to the reproductive organs of either a man or a woman. It can stop a man from being able to become a father or a woman from being able to have a baby.

What are the symptoms of syphilis?

The symptoms of syphilis are the same for both men and women. Between ten days and twelve weeks after infection a painless sore, called a *chancre*, appears on or near the sex organs. It can clearly be seen on a man's penis, but if it is inside the vagina or the rectum, the infected person may know nothing about it.

Within a few days, the sore will clear up on its own. But this does not mean the person is cured. Unless she or he has treatment, the germs will spread to other parts of the body. A few weeks later, the disease will enter its second stage, causing various symptoms such as skin rashes, mouth sores, fever, a sore throat and a general feeling of ill-health. In time, these symptoms will also disappear. The disease then enters the third stage, during which the germs continue to attack the body, but there are no apparent symptoms. This third stage can last for many years. Eventually, however, the germs severely damage every part of the body and can cause paralysis, blindness, insanity and death.

What can you do to stop yourself getting VD?

You will only catch VD by having sex with an infected person, so you can protect yourself by keeping to one sexual partner. If you have casual sex, you are putting yourself at risk. There is less risk if the man wears a condom, but the only way to be sure you won't catch VD is to avoid putting yourself at risk.

Can VD be cured?

If it is diagnosed in its early stages, VD can easily be cured by a course of suitable drugs. But the treatment does not provide you with protection against catching VD again.

Syphilis can be cured completely if it is found during the first two stages. But once it reaches the final stage, the damage that has already been done cannot be reversed. Fortunately, syphilis is not now common in Britain.

What should you do if you think you might have caught VD?

If you think you might have caught VD go either to your doctor or to a special clinic. There are special clinics at most large hospitals. You do not need an appointment or a letter from your doctor. The treatment is free and completely confidential.

AIDS

AIDS stands for Acquired Immune Deficiency Syndrome. It is a disease which damages the system by which your body protects you against infection. A person with AIDS is vulnerable to infections because an AIDS sufferer's natural immune system can no longer work properly.

What causes AIDS?

AIDS is caused by a virus called HIV. The people who are HIV positive may develop AIDS. The virus cannot survive for long outside the human body. So AIDS is not like many other infectious diseases. It cannot be spread by coughing or sneezing. You cannot catch it from sharing crockery, cutlery, or cooking utensils or from lavatory seats. Nor is AIDS a contagious disease. You cannot catch it from the casual skin contact that occurs between people in everyday life.

AIDS is spread when the virus passes directly from an infected person into another person's bloodstream. The virus can be passed on in the infected person's blood, semen or vaginal fluids during sexual activities. It can also be passed on by injection, for example, if a drug addict shares a needle and syringe with someone who is infected with AIDS.

Many haemophiliacs contracted AIDS through blood transfusions before the risk was known, but blood-screening is now so thorough that this no longer happens.

31

What are the symptoms of AIDS?

There are no immediate symptoms when a person first becomes infected with the HIV virus. The only way people can know they have become infected is when a blood test produces a positive result. But it can be up to three months after a person is infected before a blood test gives a positive result.

It is often several years after infection before the symptoms of the disease appear. During that time the person may be quite healthy, but he or she is carrying the virus and can pass it on to any sexual partner. The symptoms of AIDS vary from person to person depending on the infections they catch. The commonest symptoms include: swollen glands, profound fatigue, unexpected weight loss, fever and nightly sweats, diarrhoea, prolonged shortness of breath and a dry cough and skin disease. Once the disease has developed, most AIDS sufferers die within two to three years because they are not immune to infection.

Not everyone who is infected with the virus goes on to develop the disease. At present, there is no way of telling which people who are carrying the virus will go on to develop the disease.

Can AIDS be cured?

There is no cure at present for AIDS, though some drugs are being tried which appear to slow down the rate at which the disease develops. There is no vaccine you can be given to prevent you from getting AIDS, but research to find a vaccine is going on in many countries.

How can you protect yourself from getting AIDS?

The more sexual partners you have, the more risk there is of you coming into contact with someone who is infected. So the safest thing to do is to stick to one partner. If you do take risks, then the man should wear a condom. Using a condom won't give you one hundred per cent protection, but it cuts down the chances of your getting infected. Also, if you inject, do not share needles and syringes.

Questions

1 Why is it more difficult for a woman to tell that she has VD than it is for a man?
2 If a friend told you in confidence that she or he may have caught VD what would you say to try to persuade her or him to go to a special clinic?
3 How is AIDS spread?
4 Why is AIDS such a serious disease?
5 What activities increase a person's chances of catching AIDS?
6 Do you think the government's campaign to warn people about the dangers of AIDS has been effective?

What further questions about VD and AIDS do you want to have answered? Invite an expert such as a doctor or health education officer to come and talk to your group. Before the expert's visit, organise a question box into which people can put anonymously the questions they would like to ask.

Food hygiene

Preservation, storage and cooking.

Preserving and storing food properly keeps it from spoiling and from poisoning your body. Keeping food clean and cooking it helps to prevent germs from getting into your body.

Food poisoning

Food poisoning is caused by eating contaminated food. Food can become contaminated if it is not stored properly, if it is not cooked properly, if it is not handled properly and if the kitchen is not kept clean.

The symptoms of food poisoning vary from a mild headache to vomiting and diarrhoea. The people most at risk from food poisoning are babies and old people because they have less resistance than other people. Up to 50 deaths a year in the United Kingdom are caused by food poisoning.

Food decay

Most foods start to decay within a few days, so they must either be eaten while they are fresh or stored carefully to keep them fresh. The reasons why foods start to decay are as follows:

1 Most foods contain water which will gradually evaporate the longer the food is left exposed to the air.
2 Bacteria and other tiny organisms, such as yeast and moulds, live in many foods. They multiply rapidly, especially in warm temperatures and cause the foods to rot.
3 Chemicals, known as enzymes, which are present in foods, gradually react with other chemicals in the food and cause decay. For example, enzymes cause fruit to ripen, then if it is left uneaten they cause the fruit to decay.

How temperature affects food decay

The bacteria and enzymes which cause food decay are affected by different temperatures. If foods are heated to boiling point, most of the bacteria and enzymes are killed. At very low temperatures the bacteria and enzymes stop growing. At 5°C they grow only very slowly and at freezing point or below they hardly grow at all.

Preserving foods

Drying Many foods, including meat, can be preserved by drying the food to remove the water in it. Bacteria need water, so they cannot live and grow in dried food, and the chemical reactions which cause food to decay cannot take place without water. Drying allows you to preserve foods for months or years without having to store it in any special conditions.

Canning and bottling Lots of foods can be preserved by storing them in sealed cans or bottles. The food is mixed with water and boiled to kill the bacteria and enzymes which cause food decay. It is put in an air-tight container so that no air or germs can get in. Many foods stored in this way can be kept for several years, but when the can is opened the food must be used soon afterwards.

Freezing You can keep food fresh for several days in a refrigerator. Many foods can be preserved for longer periods by freezing them. Freezing does not kill the bacteria, but it stops them growing. When the food is thawed, the bacteria start to grow again, so frozen foods must be cooked thoroughly before you eat them.

How long you can store foods in a freezer depends on the temperature inside the freezer and the type of food you are storing. Recommended maximum storage times for most foods in star-rated freezers are shown below:

STORAGE INSTRUCTIONS	
FOOD FREEZER	★★★★ 3 MONTHS
STAR MARKED FROZEN COMPARTMENT OF REFRIGERATOR	★★★ 3 MONTHS ★★ 1 MONTH ★ 1 WEEK
REFRIGERATOR OR OTHER COOL PLACE	24 HOURS
DO NOT REFREEZE ONCE THAWED	

Foods stored in a freezer must be properly wrapped to stop the surface of the food drying out because of water loss.

Storing food

When you buy chilled or frozen foods, you should take them home and put them in the fridge or freezer as soon as possible. All foods should spend as little time as possible at temperatures between 5°C and 63°C because at these temperatures bacteria can grow rapidly. The longer you leave food in a warm car, the more chance bacteria have of starting to grow.

You should cover any raw meat and put it on the bottom shelf of the fridge. Raw meat always contains some bacteria and is likely to drip. If you put it on the bottom shelf, it won't contaminate any other food by dripping on it. The smaller the piece of meat, the sooner it decays. Mince should either be frozen or cooked straight away.

Cooking food

Heating food often softens it and makes it easier to chew and digest. It also kills off the bacteria which can cause food poisoning. Foods which need very careful cooking are meat, meat products and poultry because these foods are responsible for about two-thirds of food poisoning outbreaks.

The bacteria in whole meat joints will be on or near the surface. If the joint is roasted, the outside of the meat gets hot enough to kill the bacteria. But the bacteria on rolled joints and poultry may be deep in the flesh or joint, so the heat has to penetrate right through the flesh to reach them. This is unlikely to happen if the rolled joint or poultry is cooked straight from frozen, so it must be defrosted first. Pork joints must be thoroughly cooked all the way through in case of tape-worm infestation. Sausage meat should not be used to stuff poultry, as it may not cook properly.

Questions

1 What are the symptoms of food poisoning?
2 What are the reasons why foods start to decay?
3 How can you preserve food by
    a) drying it
    b) canning it?
4 Why does freezing food keep it fresh?
5 For how long can you store food in
    a) a refrigerator
    b) a freezer?
6 It is important to keep chilled food chilled and frozen food frozen. Why?
7 Why should you store raw meat on the bottom shelf of the refrigerator?
8 Why do we cook most of our food before eating it?
9 Why is it important to ensure that rolled joints and poultry are cooked right through?

Tasks

1 Some foods can be put straight into a freezer, others need to be prepared by *blanching* them. Explain what blanching is and how to do it. Make lists of foods you can put straight into a freezer and foods that need blanching.
2 Packets of frozen foods usually have a star-rating on them to show how long you can keep them. Study the labels on a number of frozen food packets, then draw a chart to show how long you can keep different foods for.

Hygiene in the kitchen

High standards of cleanliness are essential in the kitchen in order to prevent food from getting contaminated. If you do not take the necessary precautions, bacteria can easily get transferred onto the food you are going to eat while you are preparing it.

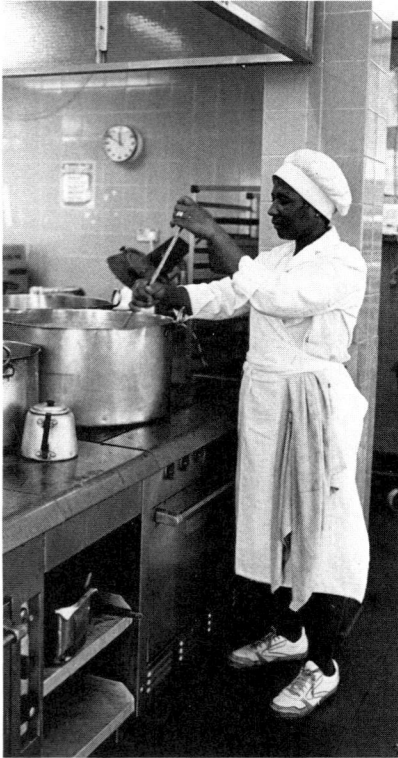

Hygiene in the kitchen is important to protect food from contamination.

Personal hygiene

The main way food gets contaminated is from unwashed hands. You should always wash your hands in hot, soapy water before starting to prepare food. Wash your hands, too, after every visit to the lavatory. Otherwise bacteria from your bowel could get onto your food. If you do not keep your fingernails clean, bacteria from dirt under your fingernails could contaminate food.

If you cut yourself, you should immediately cover the wound with a clean, waterproof dressing. This will prevent any germs from the wound getting onto the food you are handling as well as preventing any germs from getting into the wound.

It can be tempting to want to taste the food you are preparing. But you should resist the temptation to dip a finger in the food and then lick it, since you might transfer bacteria from your mouth to the food. For the same reason, you should avoid smoking, spitting, sneezing and coughing while you are working in the kitchen.

Another way you can transfer bacteria onto food is from your hair. You should not comb your hair or powder your nose in the kitchen. If your hair is long, you should tie it back.

The more you handle food directly, the more likely you are to contaminate it. Whenever possible, use forks, spoons, slices or tongs rather than your hands when you are preparing food.

Food hygiene

Food should be either eaten at once or put away, rather than be left lying around in a warm kitchen. If cooked food is to be stored, it should be cooled rapidly. Cooked meat should not be stored alongside raw meat.

If you are reheating food, you must heat it thoroughly since reheating won't destroy germs unless the heat penetrates sufficiently. It is not advisable to reheat food more than once.

Food should always be kept covered so that it will not pick up any germs from the air or from insects, such as flies. It should be stored in the refrigerator if possible or on a cool shelf, and it should not be kept for too long. If you think you might have kept some food for too long, don't risk getting food poisoning by eating it. The golden rule is 'if in doubt, throw it out'.

Kitchen hygiene

Germs can thrive in the warm moist conditions found in the kitchen. So the golden rule when working in the kitchen is

'Clear up as you go'. If you wipe the work surface down as soon as you've finished a job, it not only stops germs spreading but makes preparing the food easier. For the same reasons, you should mop up any spills as soon as they occur.

Dishcloths Nothing spreads more germs about in the kitchen than a dirty dishcloth or a dirty sponge. Dishcloths and sponges need regular washing and boiling or soaking in disinfectant. If they are used for washing up, they should not be used for anything else.

Before you wash dishes, any leftover scraps should be scraped into the bin so they don't end up in the washing-up water. Rinsing dishes in hot water after you have washed them is more hygienic than using a tea-towel which is not changed often enough.

Chopping boards All kitchen utensils should be cleaned each time they are used, especially chopping boards, because they are used for a wide range of foods including meat, fish and poultry. You can remove any bacteria by frequent scrubbing and careful drying.

Pedal bins and dustbins You should use plastic bin liners or wrap leftover food in paper before putting it in the bin. The bin should be covered to keep out flies and should be disinfected regularly.

Cupboards and floors If kitchen cupboards and the kitchen floor are not cleaned regularly, germs will start to grow on any spilt food. The floor should be washed once a week with a disinfectant solution. Cupboards should be wiped thoroughly and left to dry before any food is put back in them.

Questions

1 Why is cleanliness so important in the kitchen?
2 What advice about personal hygiene in the kitchen would you give to a friend about to start work experience in a canteen?
3 Why shouldn't you store cooked meat next to raw meat?
4 Explain what is meant by the golden rule: 'If in doubt, throw it out'.
5 What is the most hygienic way to wash dishes?
6 Explain why dishcloths should be boiled regularly.
7 Why is it necessary to clean chopping boards thoroughly each time you use them?
8 Which do you think is more important in the fight against food poisoning: strong disinfectants or a refrigerator? Give your reasons.

Task

Design a poster 'Cleanliness Matters' giving advice on the do's and don'ts of kitchen hygiene.

Environmental hazards

The air you breathe and the environment which surrounds you can damage your health if they are unclean.

Air pollution

Each day you breathe in about 14 000 litres of air. If the air is polluted it can damage your lungs or cause heart diseases.

Smoke The smoke produced by burning fires in homes and power stations can pollute the air, making it poisonous to breathe. In 1952, about 4000 people died when smoke and fog combined to produce a poisonous smog over London. Smoke pollution is now controlled by the Clean Air Acts which have created smokeless zones where only smokeless fuels can be used.

Traffic fumes Exhaust fumes from petrol engines in motor vehicles contain about 1000 toxic elements, including the poisonous gases carbon monoxide and nitrogen oxides. Many cars in Britain also use petrol to which lead has been added. The exhaust fumes contain tiny particles of lead which is very poisonous. Evidence shows that very small levels of lead in your blood can affect your brain and nervous system. In particular, it is thought to affect children's ability to concentrate and to learn.

Vehicles with diesel engines produce less air pollution because their exhaust fumes are cleaner. However, research has linked the increased use of diesel engines to an increase in the number of people suffering from asthma.

Dust Dust is a major cause of work-related illnesses. Diseases caused by dust have affected hundreds of thousands of people, often shortening their lives after a lifetime spent working in dusty conditions. For example, flour and cereal dust has caused thousands of cases of asthma among millers and bakery workers, and asbestos dust has been responsible for thousands of deaths.

Dust is dangerous because it can cause lung damage such as bronchitis, emphysema, pneumoconiosis, asthma or even cancer. The nose and throat can be affected with colds and other infections, or even nasal cancer. Skin can be damaged, leading to dermatitis, ulcers and skin cancer. Eye damage, including conjunctivitis, can result from dust pollution. Internal damage can result, including damage to the brain and nervous system, blood disorders, stomach cancer, liver and kidney disease, or bladder cancer.

Domestic animals Many people suffering from asthma are allergic to cats and dogs, as their coats carry dust, mites and sometimes fleas. The faeces of dogs pollute parks, gardens and public footpaths, and can lead to serious infections in children who play in the neighbourhood.

1 Explain what the Clean Air Acts are and why they were passed.
2 a) In many countries the sale of petrol with lead added is banned. Why?
   b) What plans does the government have for introducing lead-free petrol in Britain?
   c) Do you think lead-free petrol should be made compulsory in Britain now? Give reasons.
3 If you work in dusty conditions, what should you do to protect
   a) your lungs
   b) your eyes
   c) your skin from being damaged by the dust?
4 Why is asbestos so dangerous? How can you recognise asbestos products? What safety precautions should you take if you are working with asbestos?

Task

The local authority is responsible for protecting people from health hazards and the effects of pollution. How serious a problem is air pollution in your area? How much does your local council spend on environmental health and pollution control? Find out about the work of the Environmental Health Officer.

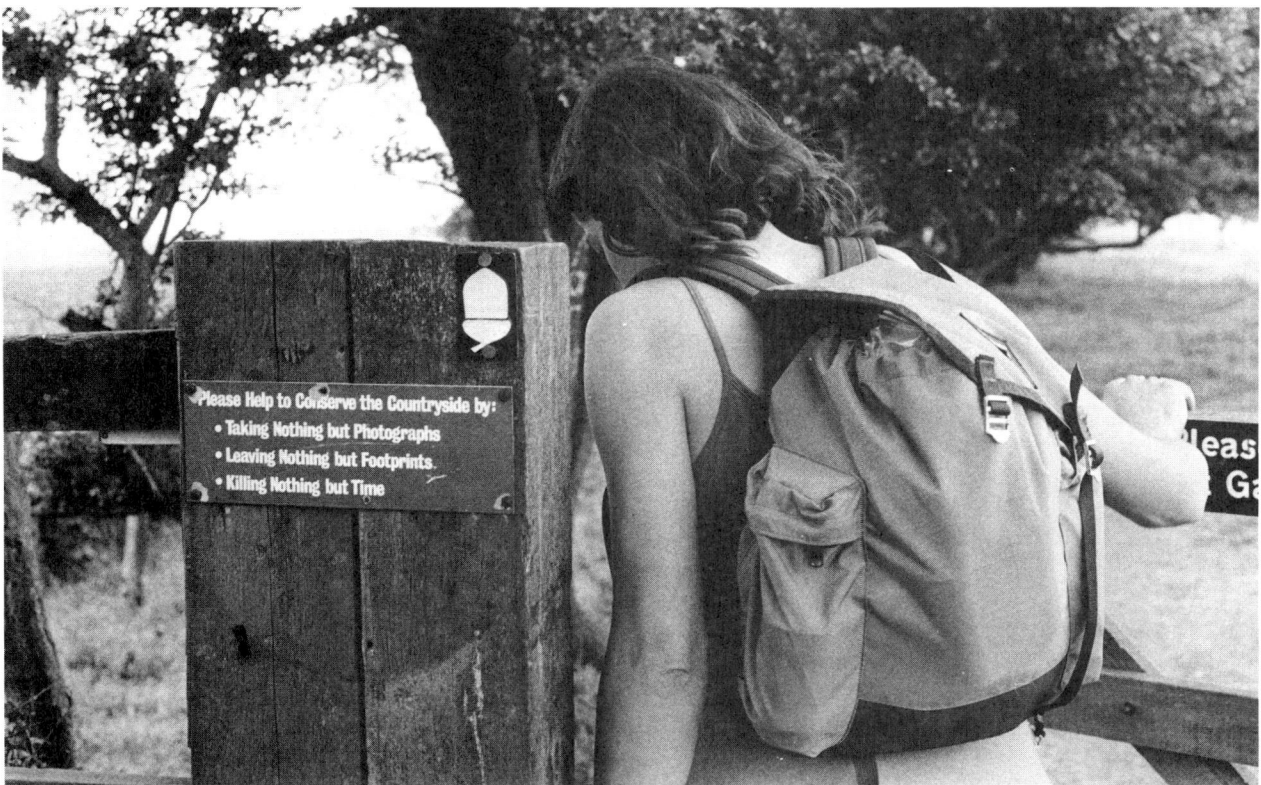

We all need to help conserve our environment.

Toxic wastes

Many industries produce chemical wastes which are highly toxic. The disposal of toxic wastes is controlled by the Deposit of Poisonous Wastes Act and the Control of Pollution Act. Dumping is forbidden except on licensed sites.

Wastes are now often taken to waste management sites. At the waste management site the wastes are either burnt or processed to make them as harmless as possible before they are dumped. Toxic wastes are transported in huge tankers. Each tanker has to meet strict safety standards and to display a card stating what chemicals it is carrying and how dangerous they are.

Radiation

The explosion at the nuclear power station at Chernobyl in Russia in 1986 showed the danger to the environment from radiation. The radioactive cloud from the explosion caused increased radioactivity 2000 kilometres from Chernobyl and in 20 countries.

Radiation causes damage to living cells and can cause death from radiation sickness and from cancer. The accident at Chernobyl showed the risks if strict safety procedures are not followed at a nuclear power station.

Radioactive wastes

Nuclear power stations produce radioactive waste which has to be stored until it is safe. High-level radioactive waste remains radioactive for thousands of years. Most high-level radioactive wastes are acids which are processed into glass blocks to guard against spillage. The blocks are then packed into special canisters. People disagree about whether it would be safer to store the canisters on land or under the sea.

Questions

1 What are toxic wastes?
2 How is the disposal of toxic wastes controlled?
3 Why is radiation so dangerous?
4 Why is the disposal of nuclear wastes a problem?

Safety in the Home

Accidents can happen anywhere, either to you or to someone nearby. Many accidents happen in the home. You need to try to prevent them and to know what to do in an emergency.

Falls

Falls are the commonest type of accidents in the home. Almost half of the injuries to children at home which require hospital treatment are the result of falls. Elderly people are more vulnerable to falls because many of them find it harder to balance and to move around steadily and they may have poor eye-sight. Even a minor fall may cause a fracture because old people's bones are more brittle.

What to do if someone falls

- Even if you think a bone is broken, do not move the person if the injury looks serious. This is particularly important if you think the neck or spine is injured because damage to the spinal cord can cause permanent paralysis.
- Go and call an ambulance.
- Keep the person warm.
- Do not give the injured person anything to drink in case she/he needs to be given an anaesthetic later.

Preventing falls

Stairs and hallways are particularly dangerous places. Floors and floor coverings need to be properly fitted and must be in good repair. There is nothing more dangerous than a worn stair carpet that is loosely fitted or a loose mat at the foot of the stairs or behind the front door.

To protect young children, fit a safety gate at the top and bottom of the stairs and board up any bannisters or railings that they might fall through. To protect old people, fit a handrail on the stairway and provide good lighting with two-way switches in the hallway and on the landing. Make sure no one leaves anything lying about on the stairs for someone to trip over.

The bath is a potential hazard for old people. A rubber mat will prevent them from slipping and a firm rail gives them something to steady themselves with as they climb in and out.

Tasks

1 The four groups most at risk from falls are babies, toddlers, do-it-yourself enthusiasts and old people. Suggest why.
2 Draw up a list of safety rules for do-it-yourself enthusiasts to advise them how to protect themselves against falls.
3 If someone is badly injured in a fall you should not move them or give them anything to drink. Explain why.

Broken bones

Sometimes when a bone is broken you can see the broken end of the bone. This is called an open fracture. It happens quite often with the shin-bone because the bone is near the surface of the skin. But if it is a closed fracture, it may be difficult to tell for certain whether a bone is broken. Signs are as follows:

- pain and tenderness at the point of injury
- swelling
- deformity or unusual shape (for example, if a leg is broken, the foot may have fallen sideways)
- loss of movement (the casualty cannot move the injured part normally)

First aid for fractures

Do not move the casualty until you have immobilised the fracture. Movement of the broken ends can cause more damage, pain and shock. If it is a broken leg, immobilise it by putting some soft padding between the legs and tying the injured leg gently but firmly to the other leg at the ankles and knees. If it is a broken arm, immobilise it by putting the casualty's arm across the chest and supporting it with an arm sling.

Cuts

About 4000 children a year need hospital treatment for cuts caused by glass. The commonest type of accident is falling through glass in a window or door. You can protect against such accidents by using safety glass, by putting polyester plastic safety film on the glass and by avoiding having glass panels in dangerous places, such as at the foot of the stairs.

First aid for cuts

If you lose too much blood your body won't get enough oxygen. Severe bleeding can cause death, so the first thing you must do is stop the bleeding. Put your thumb and/or fingers on the wound and press firmly. If it is a large cut, try pressing the edges together. Keep pressing until the bleeding stops. This may take up to 15 minutes.

If direct pressure won't stop the bleeding, press gently but firmly above and below the wound. If you can, raise the injured part so that it is above the level of the casualty's chest. This slows down the blood flow from the heart to the injured part.

A large cut which won't stop bleeding or which has gaping edges may need stitches. Don't try to clean it or to take out any object embedded in the wound. Removing it could cause more damage and might increase the bleeding, since the object may be plugging the wound. Bandage the wound with a clean dressing and get medical help.

If it is a small cut or a graze, clean the wound with soap and water, then dry it and put on a sterile dressing or an adhesive plaster. The size of the pad touching the wound must always be larger than the wound. Don't use any creams or ointments. They do not help and may delay healing by making the skin soggy.

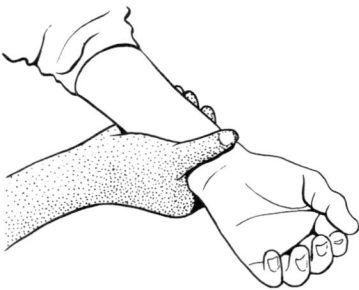

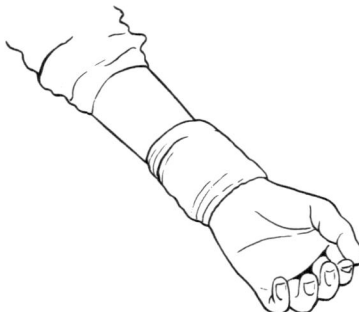

Apply pressure to stop bleeding in cuts. Bandage with a sterile dressing or adhesive plaster.

Tasks

1 List the signs and symptoms which indicate that a casualty might have a fractured leg.
2 Explain the first aid treatment you would give someone you suspected has
   a) a broken leg
   b) a broken arm.

3 What is the difference between an arm sling and an elevation sling? (Look in a First Aid Manual.)
4 If someone is bleeding badly, why is it dangerous? How would you try to stop the bleeding?
5 How would you treat
   a) a wound with an object embedded in it
   b) a grazed knee?

Burns

When you get a burn, it damages your skin and destroys the blood vessels just below the surface. The seriousness of a burn often depends on how large an area of skin has been damaged rather than on how deep the burn is.

Burns aren't just caused by fires. Many children's burns are the result of touching something hot such as an iron or an electric fire. So it is important never to leave an iron switched on or to put a hot iron in a place where a child can reach it. Always put a fire guard in front of a fire and keep children away from hot ovens and cookers. Hot dishes can be dangerous too. Always put them out of reach.

Fire hazards in the home

Every year thousands of homes are badly damaged by fire. Most of these fires are the result of carelessness.

Cigarettes and matches Many fires are caused by cigarettes or by leaving matches in places where children can find them and start to play with them. Smoking in bed is particularly dangerous.

Chip pans Lots of kitchen fires are caused by chip pans catching fire, often because the pan is too full. If a chip pan catches fire, switch the cooker off, cover the pan with a lid or a damp cloth and leave it to cool down.

Electric wiring and points Faulty electric wiring can cause a fire, as can overloading a socket by running too many appliances from it. If a socket is overloaded, the wires can overheat and start a fire.

Fires and heaters Portable fires and paraffin heaters are very dangerous if they are put in the wrong place, where they can easily be knocked over or where they are in a draught.

Flammable liquids Flammable liquids, like petrol or paraffin, should not be kept in the house. It is important to store them where they cannot be knocked over and to make sure that the tops of the cans or bottles are always firmly on. Cleaning cloths, rags and old newspapers which have been impregnated with cleaning solutions should not be stored in a cupboard under the stairs as they are inflammable, and a fire started here would cut off the escape route.

Drying clothes It is dangerous to put clothes on a fireguard to dry or to hang them too near an electric fire. Fires can also be caused by putting cookers or heaters too near curtains, which may blow in a draught and catch alight.

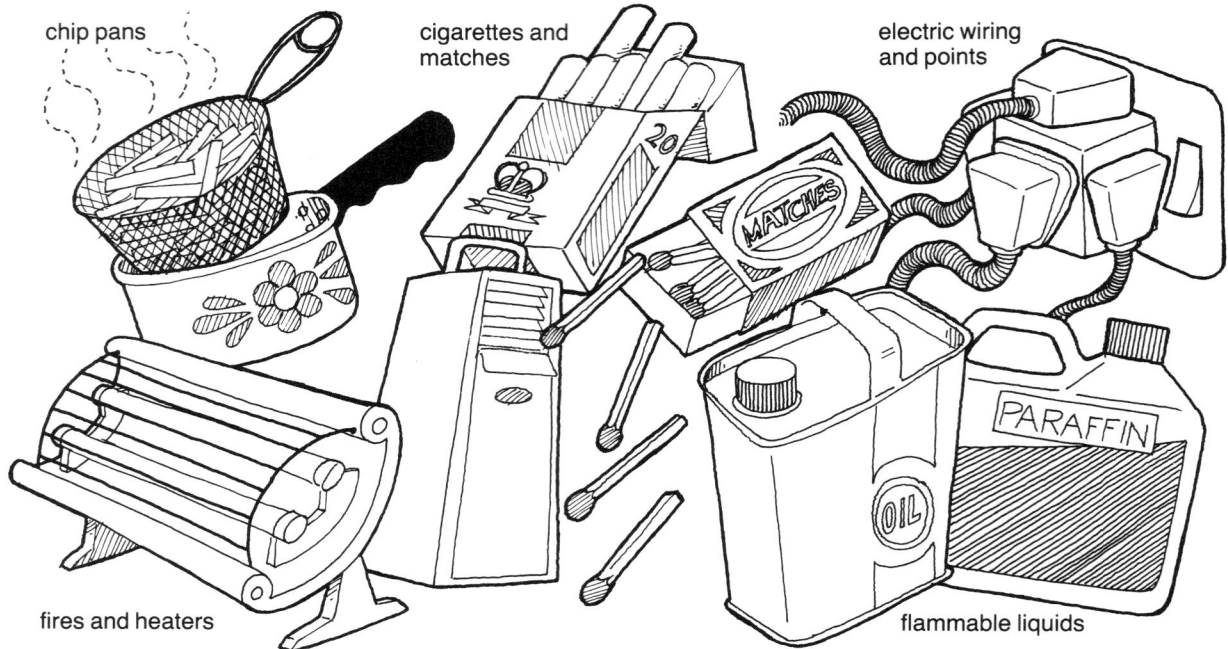

Many potential fire hazards are found in the home. Careless use of these can result in tragedy.

What should you do in an emergency?

If the house is on fire

1 Get everyone out of the house as fast as possible. Lots of deaths in fires are caused by people breathing in fumes and suffocating. So don't stay in the house and try to put the fire out.
2 Call the fire brigade by dialling 999. Don't just think that someone else will already have done so.
3 If you have time, close all doors and windows. This can stop the fire spreading, because it reduces draughts which may fan the flames.

If someone's clothes are on fire

1 Pull the person onto the ground. This stops the fire from spreading upwards towards the face.
2 Grab a coat, rug or blanket and use it to smother the flames. But don't use anything made of nylon, because nylon shrivels and melts in heat.

If someone is burned

1 Pour cold water over the burn at once. This reduces the heat in the skin.
2 Keep putting cold water on the burns for at least ten minutes. Either hold the burn under a cold tap or dip it into a bowl or a bath of cold water.

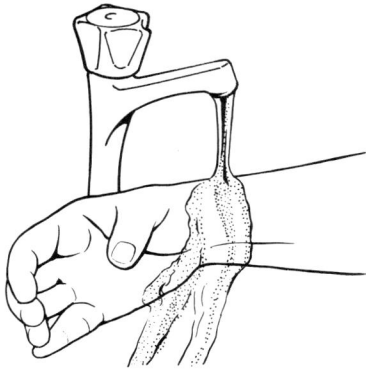

3 Burnt skin often swells up. Take off anything near the burn that may be tight such as a ring, a bracelet or a watch.

4 Cover the burn with a clean dry dressing from your first aid box or use a cotton pillow case or a linen tea towel. This will help to protect the skin from the risk of infection.

5 If the person is badly burned, call an ambulance.

6 Don't try to pull off any clothes that are stuck to the skin. Don't put any cream or ointment on the burn or use a fluffy cloth to cover the burn.

Cool a burn or scald immediately for at least ten minutes. Cover with a clean, dry dressing.

Tasks

1 Make two fire safety checklists: How to protect your home from fire.
   a) Things you should always do
   b) Things you should never do

2 You were baby-sitting when a young child got burned. Tell a friend how you gave the child first aid.

3 Design a poster either to give people advice on how to protect their homes from fire or to tell them what action to take in an emergency if a house catches fire or if someone is burned.

4 Do you know how to work a fire extinguisher? Draw a picture of one. Label its main parts. Explain in your own words how to make it work. Find out about different types of fire extinguishers and what they are used for.

Scalds

Scalds can be caused either by hot liquids or by steam. Many scalding accidents happen when young children are in the kitchen while washing or cooking is being done. If a kettle flex is left dangling or a pan handle is left sticking out, a young child can reach up and pull them over. When you are cooking or making a cup of tea or coffee, put a baby in a playpen. Other dangers include the following:

Hot drinks You should never leave a hot drink where a child might knock it over or put a child on your lap while you are having a hot drink.

Table-cloths You should avoid using a table-cloth that a child might pull at. If you put anything hot like a teapot on a table covered by a cloth, tuck the edges under the cloth instead of leaving them hanging down.

Bathroom When you are filling a bath, you should always put the cold water in first. Then add the hot water and test its temperature before putting a young child in. The water should be comfortably warm rather than hot. The temperature of the water does not have to be very high before it will scald a young child. The hot water system should be kept at a temperature which is not high enough to cause scalding. A baby or toddler should not be left alone in the bath in case he or she is tempted to try to turn the hot tap on.

1 Explain how scalding accidents can occur
   a) in the kitchen
   b) in the bathroom.
2 Why are the victims of scalding accidents often young children?
3 Suggest why scalding accidents are more likely to happen to old people than to younger adults.
4 The first aid treatment for scalds is the same as the treatment for burns (see pages 44-45). Explain why:
   a) You should put cold water on the scald for at least ten minutes.
   b) You should remove anything tight such as a belt or a wristwatch.
   c) You should cover the scald with a clean dry piece of cloth or dressing.
   d) You should not put butter, oil or ointment on a scald.
   e) You should not prick any blisters.

Suffocation and choking

Babies are most at risk from suffocation and choking. But accidents can also happen to older children when they are left playing on their own.

Suffocation

Suffocation may be caused by fumes, a plastic bag or something tight round the neck or over the face. A baby should have her own cot which is made to an approved safety design. So when you are buying a cot, you should look for the British Standards Kitemark on the label. You shouldn't use a pillow in a cot, since a baby can easily suffocate on a pillow.

Babies can get ribbons twisted round their necks. So ribbons on clothes and dummies should be kept short. Another danger is open weave clothes and cardigans with cords or ribbons threaded through the neck. If they catch on a pram or cot, they can pull tight around the neck. A baby sleeping in a pram or cot should be protected by a net over the hood, as cats attracted by the warmth might sleep on its face.

A plastic bag pulled over the head cuts off the air supply and causes suffocation. Do not leave plastic bags lying around where children might start playing with them.

If someone is suffocating, quickly remove what is causing the suffocation. If the person has stopped breathing, give mouth to mouth resuscitation.

Choking

Babies should never be left alone when they are feeding. If you leave a baby propped up alone with a bottle, the baby can easily choke.

Babies put things in their mouths to find out what they are like. If they swallow small objects such as buttons or coins they can choke. When there is a baby in the house, you must be careful not to leave small objects within their reach.

Examine carefully any toys you give them to see whether there are things like glass eyes, which the baby might pull out and put in her mouth. Avoid giving young children peanuts. There have been lots of cases of young children choking on peanuts.

If a baby chokes

1 Don't bother trying to pull the object out with your fingers. The chances are it will be too slippery and too far back. You may end up pushing the obstruction further down the throat and you will have wasted vital time.
2 Hold the baby by the legs and turn her upside down. Slap her firmly on the back between the shoulder blades several times until the object comes out.
3 If this doesn't work, give a short sharp squeeze on the baby's tummy. This should force the object up out of the baby's windpipe.
4 If you can't get the object out, treat it as an emergency and call an ambulance.

If an adult chokes while eating

1 Remove any food or false teeth from the mouth.
2 Bend the person over so that the head is lower than the lungs. Using the heel of your hand, give them four slaps between the shoulder blades.
3 If this does not dislodge the food, stand behind the person and put one arm round their middle. Clench your fist with your thumb inwards between the breastbone and the tummy button. Put your other arm round them, hold the clenched fist with your other hand and give a short, sharp squeeze. Continue giving squeezes until the food is forced up out of the windpipe.

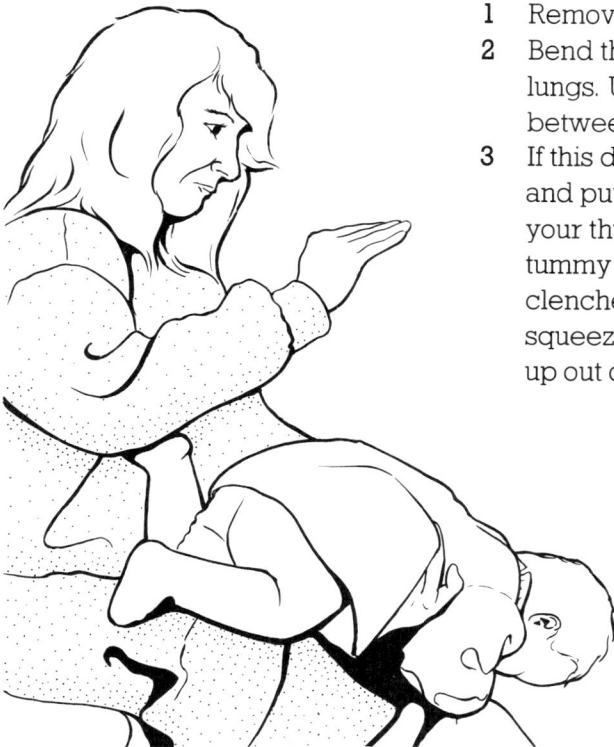

If slapping does not dislodge an obstruction, give a short squeeze on the baby's tummy.

Questions

1 Why are babies more at risk of suffocating and choking than other people?
2 Suggest the types of accident that might cause suffocation when young children are playing on their own.
3 Draw a series of diagrams to illustrate how to give first aid to
   a) a choking baby
   b) an adult who chokes while eating.

Pills and medicines

It is tragic also that medicines, prescribed to restore health, should so often be the cause of accidental poisoning. Most poisoning accidents are caused by careless use or failure to follow the instructions.

Your medicine can be a child's poison

Hundreds of people die every year from accidental poisoning. Tens of thousands more are admitted to hospital. The careless storage and use of medicines is one of the most frequent causes of these accidents.

Young children, particularly those aged from two to ten, are at special risk. Every child puts things into its mouth. Food, fingers, fluff from the teddy bear, coal from the scuttle and sweets from the box are all something to lick or suck. For the toddler there are drawers, bed-side tables, cupboards and handbags to explore.

To children brightly coloured tablets and capsules are exactly like sweets – just the right size and shape for sucking and swallowing.

The result: accidental poisoning sends young children into hospitals in increasing numbers every year – and sometimes to the mortuary.

These needless tragedies can be avoided by observing a few common-sense rules:

1   Keep all medicines out of the reach of children.
2   Store medicines in the home in a proper medicine cabinet with a safety locking device (preferably made to the British Standard specified) and close it tightly after use.
3   Never let a child play with medicine containers, empty or full.

When you are giving or taking medicines

1   Always read directions carefully and give or take the exact dose recommended.
2   Always follow the doctor's instructions. Often the doctor will give you a course of medicine to take. You should go on taking the medicine for the length of time the doctor said, even if you start to feel better much earlier.
3   Never give a medicine which has been prescribed to you to someone else who seems to have a similar ailment.
4   Never 'borrow' medicines that seem to be the same as yours.
5   Never take or give medicines in the dark.
6   While you are taking medicine prescribed by your doctor, do not take any other medicine without seeking her/his advice.
7   If you are giving tablets or capsules to a child, never call them sweets.
8   Do not take medicines or tablets yourself in front of young children.

9   If you are taking medicine, after each dose make a note of how much is left in the bottle.

10 Do not hoard any unused medicine. Either flush it down the lavatory or hand it in to the chemist. Never throw old medicines in the dustbin or put them on the fire.

11 Never transfer medicine to another container and never put anything else in an empty medicine bottle. Throw the bottle away or hand it back to the chemist.

12 After use, always put medicines back in the medicine cabinet and keep it locked.

If you think a child may have swallowed some pills or tablets

1   Look quickly to see if you can find the missing tablets. For example, if the container is lying empty on the floor, have the tablets rolled under a table or chair?

2   Take the child to either a doctor or a hospital – whichever is the nearest. If you know what the child has swallowed, take the empty container with you, so that the doctor will know exactly what she/he has taken.

3   Do not try to make the child sick by giving salt and water. Large amounts of salt can be very dangerous.

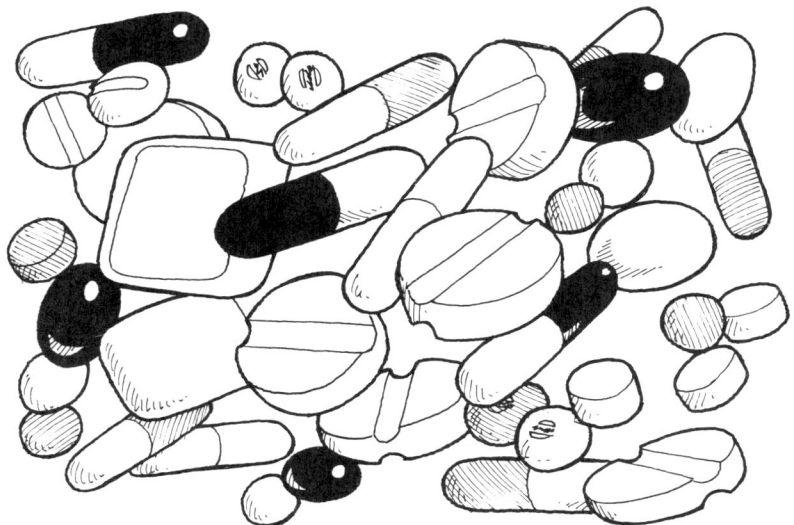

Brightly coloured tablets and capsules are sometimes mistaken for sweets by children. Keep all medicines in a safe place and never refer to medicine as 'sweets'.

Questions

1   Study the advice on how to use medicines safely and suggest reasons for each piece of advice.

2   Accidental poisonings often happen when children are visiting elderly relatives or when a relative or friend comes to stay. Suggest why. What can you do to try to prevent such accidents from happening?

3   Why are many tablets now often packed in blister or strip packs rather than in bottles?

4   Some friends with a young child are about to move into a new house. What advice would you give them about getting a medicine cabinet, what they should keep in it, where they might put it and where they should keep the key?

Household chemicals

A great risk to children are the many household chemicals that we have in our houses and garages. It is important to store them out of children's reach.

Something to get bitter about

Every day in Britain over 200 under-fives are rushed to their doctor or local hospital because they have swallowed a household chemical. The main danger zones within the home are not only the kitchen and bathroom, but also the living-room and bedroom where we keep many alcohol-based products that we don't think of as chemicals, though of course, they are. The garden shed and garage are also potential danger areas if not kept locked. It is essential to keep tubes of glue etc. out of the reach of small children; not only are they dangerous to swallow or inhale, but they sometimes need hospital treatment to remove.

Hospital records show that accidents with turpentine, bleach, disinfectant, rat poison, scent, glue, shampoo, after-shave and lavatory cleaners occur most often. Curiously, substances we think of as particularly dangerous such as bleach, disinfectant and insecticides are not very poisonous to humans. They may be good at killing germs and pests, but they don't kill children. In fact few chemicals that are designed for use around the home are capable of killing us, which is why so few accidents of this kind end in the death of the child.

Even so, medical treatment for the injuries that household chemicals cause to the mouth and throat must be obtained as quickly as possible, but there is no need to panic – these substances are not *deadly* poisons. Treatment for most cases consists chiefly of soothing medicines plus lots to drink to dilute the chemical and help the body to get rid of it naturally. Stomach pumping is rarely used by doctors, though this is popularly imagined to be the only way of dealing with accidents of this kind.

If a child swallows a harmful substance make him spit out any remaining poison but do *not* try to make him vomit. If the product was a caustic material (acid or alkali) or petroleum-based (like turps or weedkiller) give the child milk to drink. After any poisoning phone your doctor for advice or go straight to the nearest hospital accident and emergency department.

However, there are some products that we use a lot that are very dangerous. Paraffin, turpentine and turps substitute, paint stripper, caustic soda (used to unblock drains) and toiletries made from alcohol all put a toddler much more at risk. Swift action is essential, but it is still rare for a child to be detained in hospital for more than a couple of days.

This does not alter the fact that household chemicals are a source of worry. One answer to the problem has been to market them in containers sealed with child resistant caps. The use of these is a step in the right direction as long as we

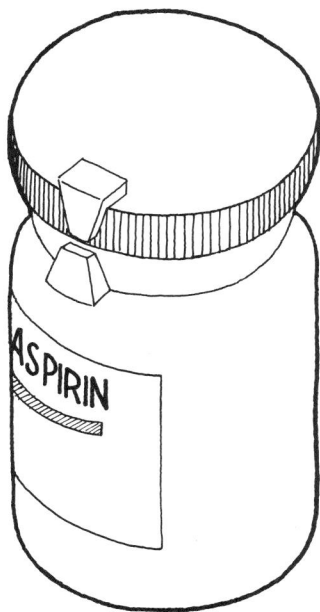

Child resistant caps have helped to reduce the number of accidental poisonings of children.

remember always to screw the top back on properly. Yet as Esther Rantzen's 'That's Life' showed, some very young children were clever enough to undo them.

Putting child resistant caps on dangerous bottles is one answer. Yet this wouldn't prevent a quarter of all accidents which involve a child drinking a chemical that has been transferred from its original container to a more convenient one. As long as we enjoy the benefits of useful chemicals in the home it seems we must pay the price of being constantly on the watch or take the consequences.

But must it be so? A better way would be to make all household chemicals *undrinkable*. This can be done by adding a repellent. Moves are afoot to add the bitterest substance known – Bitrex – to lots of them.

This material is already used to make industrial alcohol undrinkable and it is also put into anti-nail biting nail varnishes. Research with children shows it also prevents them drinking undesirable fluids. When it was tested on a relatively harmless detergent solution, children reacted to it immediately, spat it out and didn't try drinking the detergent again. Some supermarket chains such as Tesco's are now planning to add Bitrex to appropriate household products.

This extra safeguard for children is not likely to make products more expensive. Less than a thousandth of an ounce of Bitrex is needed to make a litre bottle of detergent or disinfectant too bitter to drink. But even if it added a penny to the cost of every item, it would pay for itself many times over and not just in savings for the NHS, but in preventing many of the mental traumas suffered by both parents and children.

(adapted from an article in 'Woman')

Tasks

1 List ten pieces of information about household chemicals which you learned from the article.
2 Study the labels on a number of household chemicals. Note the warnings they carry and make a chart listing them in order of how dangerous each one is starting with the most dangerous.
3 Many products are sold in pressurised containers (aerosols). What warnings are printed on aerosol cans?
4 Gardens should be places where you can relax and enjoy yourself. Yet many accidents occur in gardens. List the types of accidents that can occur in gardens. Then, draw up a list of advice on safety in the garden.
5 List the types of accidents that can occur in garages and garden sheds. Draw up a list of advice on safety in garages and garden sheds.
6 Describe what you should do if you found a child in your care had opened a bottle of bleach and has swallowed some.
7 What should a first aid kit contain? Look at the picture of the contents of a first aid box on the next page. Give a reason why each item is included and suggest five other items you might put in a first aid box. Say why they would be useful.

What to put in a first aid kit

1 Box of adhesive dressings (various sizes)
2 Box of sterile gauze dressings (various sizes)
3 Small packet of paper tissues
4 2 or 3 cotton bandages
5 2 or 3 crepe bandages
6 Triangular bandages, or clean old linen or cotton tea towel, or other cotton cloth
7 Small roll of cotton wool
8 Blunt-ended scissors
9 Safety pins and roll of adhesive tape
10 Small bar of soap
11 Antiseptic cream

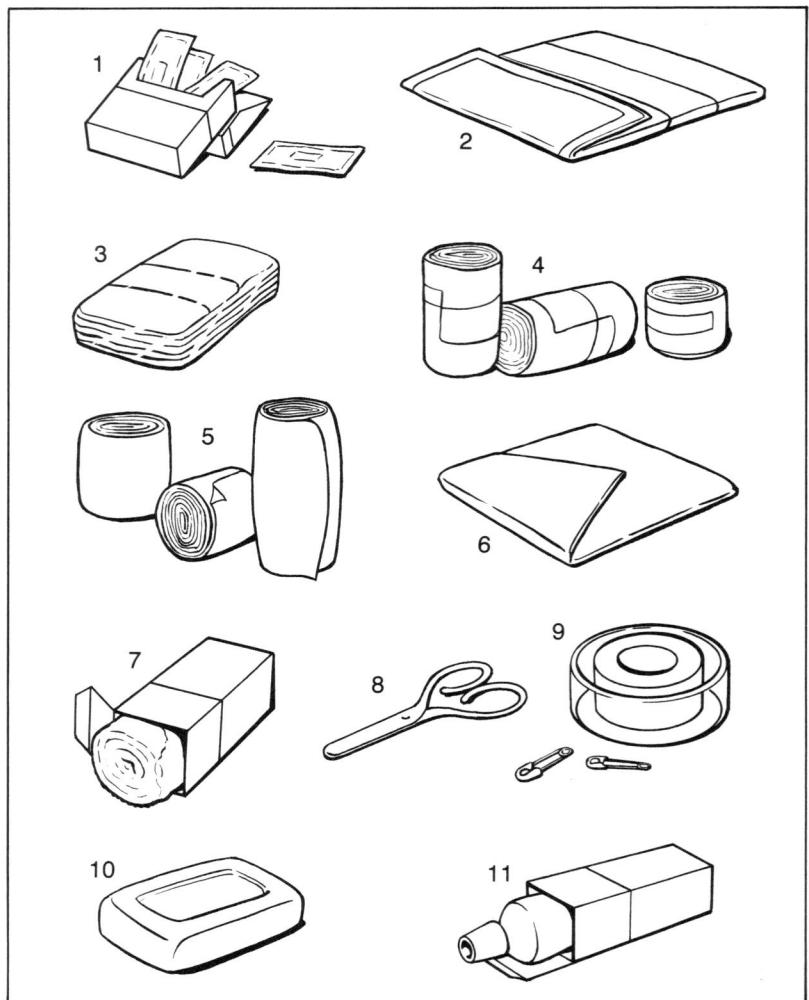

Electrical safety

Electrical appliances are a potential source of danger. Only attempt to fit plugs and replace fuses yourself. Leave other repairs to a qualified electrican.

Safety standards

When you buy new electrical goods, you can make sure that they are safe by checking that they conform to approved safety standards. Often, it is tempting to buy second-hand electrical equipment because it is cheaper. But there is no way of knowing whether or not second-hand appliances are safe.

Plugs These should have the number BS 1363 on them. This means the model of plug has been tested and conforms to British Standards. Plugs should also have the ASTA mark on them, showing that they have been approved by the Association of Short Circuit Testing Authorities.

If there are young children in the house, it is a good idea to buy plugs which have 'ears' on them because they are harder to pull out. You can also get plugs with part-insulated pins which offer more protection if children try to touch them.

Electrical goods New electrical equipment should have a BEAB safety label on it. BEAB stands for the British Electrotechnical Approvals Board. The BEAB Mark of Safety is yellow and blue. It tells you that the model you are buying has been carefully tested for its safety and conforms to approved British Standards.

Using electrical equipment safely

In the kitchen When you are working in the kitchen, you should dry your hands before using any electrical appliances. Water conducts electricity, so touching plugs or sockets with wet hands is very risky. For the same reason, you should always unplug an electric kettle before filling it.

If you are ironing, watch out for the flex. A common cause of accidents with irons is burning the flex with the hot iron. Accidents can also be caused by the flex being trailed across the cooker. Avoid letting the flex hang down where a young child can reach up and pull it. Another danger is plugging the iron into a light socket. Light circuits are not strong enough to provide the power needed by appliances such as irons.

Accidents with toasters usually happen because a piece of bread gets stuck. Someone picks up a knife or a fork and starts poking around inside the toaster, forgetting that cutlery is made of metal which conducts electricity. If a piece of bread gets stuck, you should switch off the toaster and let it cool down before you start trying to get the toast out.

In the living room TV sets use a high voltage. It is very dangerous to operate them with the back cover off. Any repairs should be carried out by a specialist engineer.

Always allow a 'dead' light-bulb to cool, and check that the light-switch is off before fitting a new bulb. Do not use a high-voltage bulb in a small shade.

Using an adaptor to run lots of appliances from the same power point can overload the house wiring: you risk starting a fire. If there are not enough power points for your needs, you should ask an electrican to fit some more sockets.

Flexes should be kept short. Long flexes are a hazard because people may trip over them. If you put a flex under a carpet or rug, it may get worn or damaged without you noticing. When a flex is damaged, you should always replace it rather than join it. If you do repair it, then use proper connectors.

In the bathroom Extra precautions are necessary in the bathroom because of the danger of using electricity where there is water. Ordinary electric sockets are not allowed in bathrooms and switches have to be pullcords. The only socket permitted is a special shaver socket.

The only appliances you should use are a shaver or an electric toothbrush. You should never use portable appliances, such as fires or hair-driers, even if they are plugged in elsewhere.

Electric lawn-mowers A number of accidents are caused by misuse of, or faults in, electric mowers and similar appliances.

1 Do not switch on power until the machine is fully connected.
2 Rake the lawn before mowing, to remove stones, twigs or other objects.
3 Wear protective (preferably rubber-soled) shoes and thick gloves.
4 Protect the eyes.
5 Do *not* allow the flex to get under the blades.
6 Switch off power before cleaning or repairing any part of the machine.
7 Have regular professional maintenance carried out on all major household or gardening equipment.

Essential safety rules

1 If a fault occurs, *Switch Off Straightaway*, then investigate the cause.
2 Call in the experts. Don't try to do repairs yourself, except to plugs, fuses and flexes.

Tasks

1 Study the pictures. What electrical safety rules are being broken in the kitchen and in the living-room? Make two lists saying what is being done wrong and what the dangers are.

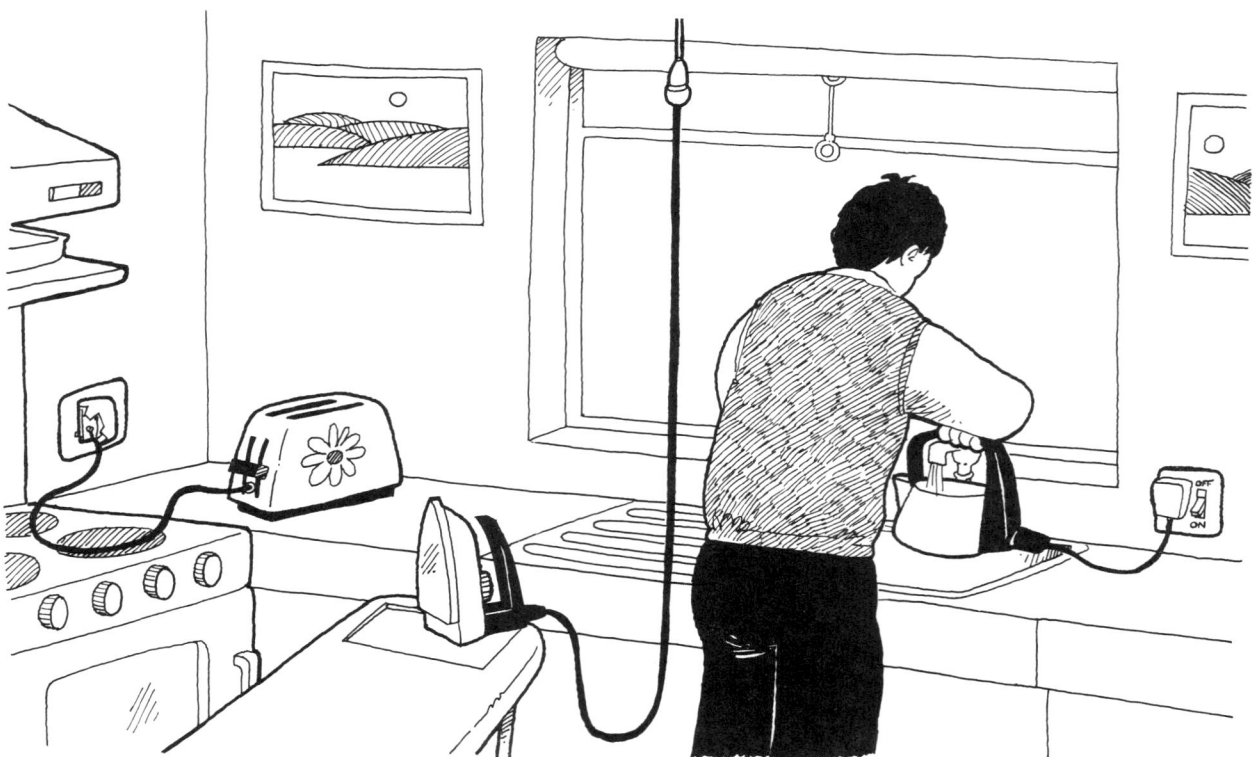

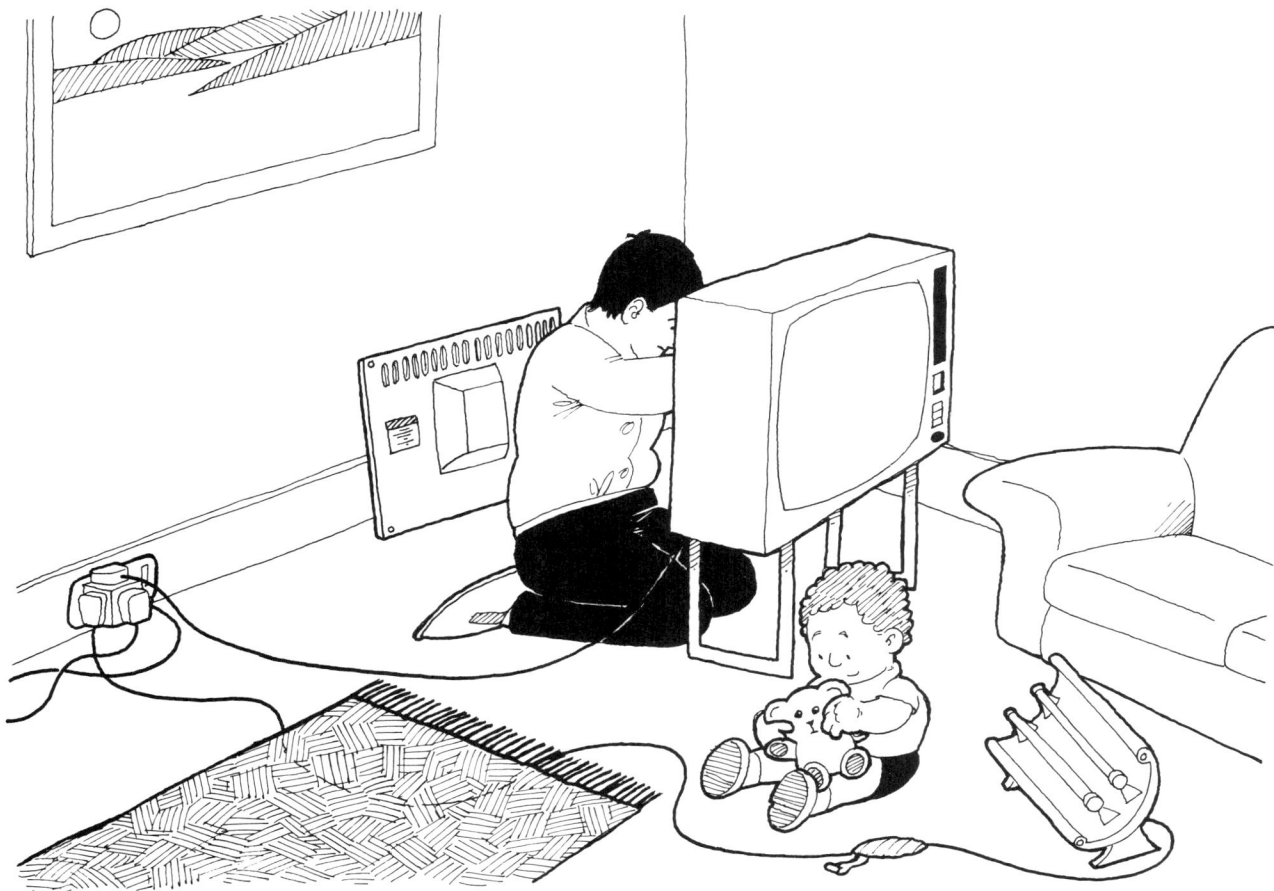

2   a) What should you always look for when buying a plug?
     b) If you have young children, which is the best type of plug to buy?

3   When you buy electrical goods, you should look for the BEAB label. What is the BEAB label? What does it tell you?

4   Write out a set of numbered instructions explaining how to carry out these electrical repairs safely:
     a) changing a fuse in a plug
     b) wiring a plug
     c) changing a fuse in the main fuse box.
     (You can find details of how to wire plugs and change fuses in the leaflet Electricity and You – Plugs and Fuses, available from your local Electricity Board or in the Lifeskills book, pages 8 to 10.)

Gas safety

There are laws and guidelines set up to protect you from danger from accidents involving gas. If you break the gas safety laws, you can be fined up to £2000.

Gas safety laws

- Gas officials have the right to enter any building to inspect the gas supply and gas appliances.
- It is your responsibility to make sure the gas appliances in your home are not dangerous.

- Gas fitting must be done by experts. You must not fit or service gas supplies or appliances yourself.
- It is your responsibility to turn off your main gas supply if you suspect there is a leak and to contact the local gas service.
- You must not turn the supply on again or use the appliance until the leak has been repaired.

If you smell gas

Gas is dangerous because it forms an explosive mixture with air. If you smell gas you should remember the following:

1 Put out any cigarettes or other naked lights. Do not strike any matches.
2 Do not switch any electric plugs or switches on or off. This could cause a spark.
3 Open windows and doors to let the gas out and leave them open until the leaking stops.
4 Check the gas taps on all your appliances to see if one has been left on and check to see if a pilot light has gone out.
5 Turn off the main gas supply at the meter. The diagrams show the on and off positions.
6 Call the gas service. The emergency number to ring is listed in the telephone directory under GAS.

Gas accidents

Natural gas is not poisonous. But the fumes from a gas fire or heater contain carbon monoxide, which is a deadly gas. So gas appliances must be properly ventilated and chimneys and flues cleaned regularly so they do not get blocked.

Gas boilers and water heaters should be serviced every year. Over half the accidents caused by faulty appliances involve appliances that were bought second-hand. Before you buy a second-hand appliance, it is worth getting expert advice.

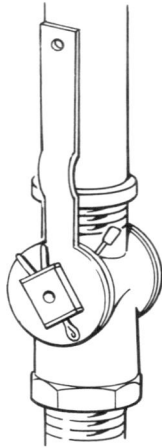

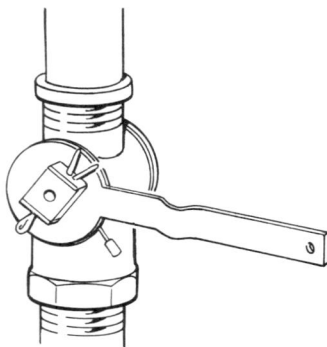

When the tap is lying along the pipe, the gas supply is on. When the tap is lying across the pipe at right angles to it, the gas supply is off.

Task

Use the information on gas safety to answer the crossword.

Clues across
1 Open these if you smell gas (5)
4 When the tap is lying in this position in relation to the pipe, the main gas supply is on (5)
7 Gas officials can do this to inspect the supply and appliances in any building (5)
8 Gas fires produce these containing carbon monoxide (5)
10 If you smell gas, check to see one has not gone out (5)
12 If you smell gas, check to see one has not been left turned on (3)
14 This makes an explosive mixture with gas (3)
15 If you smell gas, do not operate electric switches in case you cause one (5)
17 Appliances like this are more likely to be faulty than new ones (6–4)

Clues down

2 Leave windows open until a gas escape has been repaired to let the gas ... (3)

3 It is your responsibility to make .... the appliances in your home are safe (4)

5 Do not leave the gas supply like this if you think there is a leak (2)

6 Turn this off if there is a leak (3,6)

7 You must get these people to fix or service gas supplies and appliances (7)

8 You are breaking the law if you buy an appliance and do this to it yourself (3)

9 The tap for the main gas supply is usually near this (5)

11 If you suspect an appliance or a gas pipe is doing this, you must contact the gas service (7)

13 Do not use this to look for a gas leak (5)

16 Gas boilers and water heaters should be serviced every .... (4)

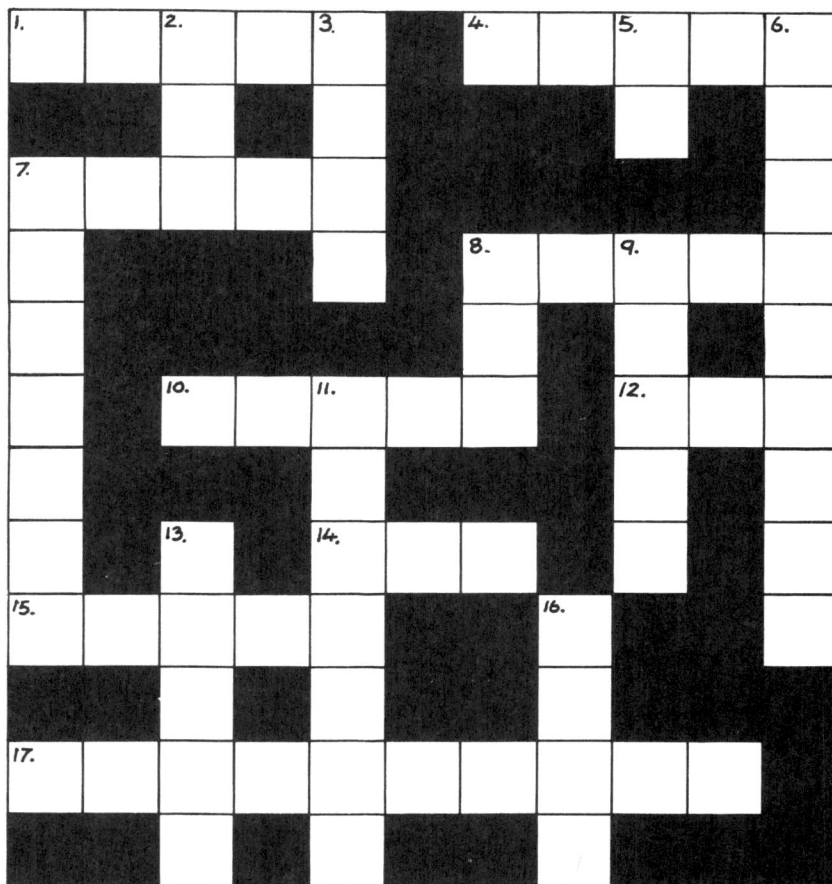

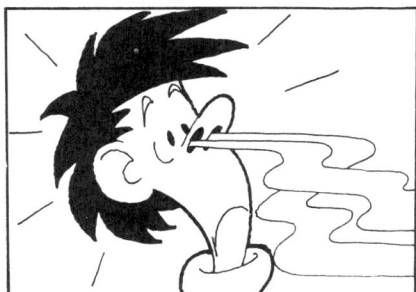

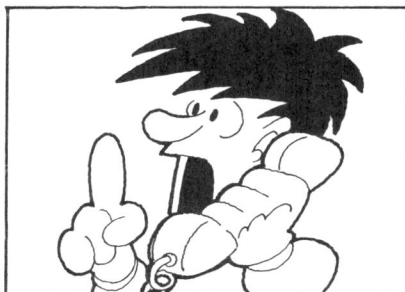

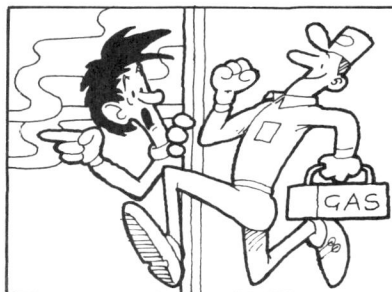

Emergency first aid

When you are faced with an emergency, do not rush in immediately with first aid. Pause to assess the situation first. Look around to make sure that you are not going to endanger yourself or the victim. You must then decide how the injury should be treated.

Unconsciousness

1   Check that the person is breathing properly. Make sure there are no obstructions in the mouth. Remove any false teeth, chewing gum or vomit.
2   Stop any severe bleeding by pressing firmly on the wound.
3   If the person stops breathing, give mouth-to-mouth resuscitation.
4   It can be dangerous for an unconscious person to lie on her or his back, because the tongue may fall back and block the airway. Once you are sure that breathing is satisfactory and any severe bleeding is controlled, you should put the person in the recovery position. This prevents the tongue from falling back and allows any blood, fluid or vomit to drain out of the mouth.
5   It can be dangerous to move someone who has broken bones or internal injuries. Do not move such a casualty unless you have to do so because there is further danger, such as from traffic or fire.
6   Do not leave an unconscious person alone unless you have to do so because there is no one else around and you need to go to fetch help.

Shock

A person who has had a serious injury, severe pain or serious loss of blood may be suffering from the condition called shock. The symptoms of shock vary depending on how serious the condition is. The symptoms include paleness, feeling faint, cold and clammy skin, a weak and fast pulse, fast and shallow breathing. Shock can cause unconsciousness and even death. The aim of first aid for shock is to prevent the shock from developing or getting worse.

1   Get the casualty to lie down and deal with any injuries.
2   If the casualty has lost a lot of blood, keep the head down and if possible raise the lower limbs. But do not do this if you think there may be a head injury or that a leg may be broken.
3   Cover the casualty with a blanket, rug or coat to keep him or her warm, but not too hot.
4   Do not give anything to drink in case the person needs to have an anaesthetic when she/he gets to hospital.

1 Draw up a list of do's and don'ts when giving emergency first aid to
   a) an unconscious person
   b) someone who is suffering from shock.
2 Study a first aid manual. Work with a partner and practise putting each other into the recovery position.

Safety on the Road

There are many dangers which you face on the road – as a pedestrian, a cyclist, a motorcyclist or in a car. You should watch out for possible dangers and try to observe good safety rules.

Pedestrians

Every year thousands of pedestrians are injured in accidents. Some of them are disabled for life. Several hundred are killed. The people most at risk are very young children and people aged over 60.

Most young children injured or killed in accidents in the street are on their own. Every time parents allow a young child out in the street unaccompanied, they are taking a risk with the child's life. Sixty per cent of accidents involving children under the age of five happen within 100 yards of the child's home.

What to do if a pedestrian gets knocked down

Keep calm, sum up the situation and decide what needs to be done.

1 Make sure there's no further danger to the injured person from any other traffic. If necessary, ask someone to control the traffic.
2 Send someone to find a phone and call an ambulance.
3 Do not attempt to move the casualty. If she is unconscious, turn her head to one side and check that the airway is not blocked so that she can breathe. Put a coat or a blanket over her to keep her warm.
4 Check to see if there is any serious bleeding. If there is, try to stop it by pressing down hard on the place it is coming from.
5 Remain with the casualty, comforting and reassuring her until the ambulance comes.

Questions

1 Suggest the reasons why the very young and the over-sixties are more at risk than other groups of people.
2 List the safest places and the most dangerous places to cross the road.

3   Write out the Green Cross Code, then check in the Highway Code to see how accurately you have remembered it.
4   What should you do if you are crossing the road at
    a) a zebra crossing
    b) a pelican crossing?
5   If you have to cross the road between parked cars, what should you do?
6   If there is no footpath, where should you walk?
7   If you are walking on the road at night, what should you do to protect yourself?
8   You are driving along the road and you see a pedestrian knocked down by a car which does not stop. What should you do:
    a) follow the car to get its number
    b) drive to a phone box and call the police
    c) stop and help the injured person? Give your reasons.

Cyclists

There is more risk of a cyclist having a road accident than any other road user except a motorcyclist. You are especially at risk on a bicycle when turning right, crossing the pavement to the road, at roundabouts and at night.

Turning right

1   Look behind you to check for traffic.
2   If it's clear, give an arm signal early.
3   Move towards the centre of the road to take up the correct position for turning.
4   Repeat the arm signal and give a last 'life-saver' look over your right shoulder before turning.

At roundabouts

You must give way to traffic coming on your right. It is usually safer to stay in the left-hand lane and to watch out for vehicles wanting to cross your path to leave the roundabout.

Crossing the pavement

Riding across the pavement and straight out into the road causes accidents in two ways: accidents involving pedestrians, accidents involving vehicles. You should wheel your bicycle across the pavement and then wait for a gap in the traffic.

At night

Riding at night is hazardous because it can be difficult for other drivers to see you in the dark. It is an offence to ride without proper lighting. The law requires you to have an efficient white light in front and a red light and a red reflector behind. What else can you do to make sure you are seen?

Tasks

1 Design a comic-strip or write a cautionary tale for young children about a youngster who ignored one of the above pieces of advice and had an accident.
2 Draw up a list of do's and don'ts for cyclists. Compare your list with the 'Extra Rules for Cyclists' in the Highway Code.
3 The most dangerous age for cyclists is 12 to 14; five times as many boys get hurt as girls. Suggest why.
4 List in order of safety the various ways of carrying things on a bicycle. Which are the safest ways and why?
5 It is a good idea to fix a spacer bar on your bicycle. Why? What other things can you
   a) fit to your bicycle
   b) wear to make cycling safer?
6 How often should you check your bicycle? Which parts should you check? Write out a bicycle maintenance schedule. (See the section on Vehicle Safety in the Lifeskills book.)

Motorcyclists

Motorcyclists are in more danger than other road users. That's because they have less protection than drivers. So whenever you go on a motorcycle, even if you are only going a short distance, always wear proper clothes.

Helmets

It is against the law to ride a motorcycle without a crash-helmet on. The helmet must be fastened. If you have a passenger, the passenger must wear a helmet too.

There are two types of crash-helmet. An open-face helmet provides protection for your skull, but not the whole of your face. So you will need to wear either goggles or a visor to protect your eyes.

A full-face helmet is safer because it provides more protection. The chin cup protects your chin and jaw and the visor protects your eyes.

Whatever type of helmet you choose, it is important to look after it properly. Do not paint it or put any stickers on it. Paint and stickers can damage some helmets and cause them to break up if you have an accident. Clean the helmet regularly using soapy water. Do not use either solvents or detergents because they might damage the helmet.

If you have an accident and your helmet is damaged, get a new one. Even if the helmet looks undamaged, get someone to check it for you. Always wear a clear visor. If your visor is scratched, buy a new one. It is dangerous to ride with a scratched visor, especially in bad weather conditions.

Gloves, boots and suits

Wear a thick pair of leather gloves to protect your hands and a strong pair of boots or shoes on your feet. Do not ride in trainers or plimsolls. They don't offer enough protection.

If you can afford it, buy a proper well-padded motorcycling suit. A leather suit is best. Get one that is not too tight-fitting. Whatever you do, do not ride a motorcycle in shorts or a T-shirt.

It takes a few extra minutes to get properly dressed for motorcycling. But it is time well spent. It can prevent you from getting badly grazed, cut or bruised if you come off.

At night-time, wear something bright so that other motorists can see you easily. Put a reflective top over your jacket or wear a reflective strip over your shoulder. Be safe – Be seen.

Motorcycle maintenance

Motorcycles must be kept in a roadworthy condition. Keep the engine clean and regularly check the brakes, the tyres and the lights.

Brakes You should check your brakes whenever you ride. As you move off, test first the front brake and then the rear brake. Keep an eye on the wear indicators, so that you can tell when the brake pads or linings need replacing.

Tyres Tyres must always have the correct amount of air in them. The correct tyre pressure is vital to make the types grip the road. Also, check your tyres for wear. If your tyres are worn, you should buy new ones at once. It is against the law to have worn tyres because they do not grip the road surface firmly enough.

Lights By law your lights and indicators must be working properly whenever you ride. Your headlight beam must be properly aligned so that it does not shine in the eyes of oncoming motorists and dazzle them.

Tasks

1 Read the advice (above) about what to wear when you ride a motorcycle.
   a) Make a list of the proper clothes to wear for motorcycling.
   b) Draw a diagram of the equipment you need for motorcycling.
   c) Explain why you should never wear trainers, shorts and a T-shirt when you are riding a motorcycle.
   d) What extra item should you wear at night? Explain why.
2 A friend cannot decide what type of helmet to buy. Write a short conversation between you and the friend in which you advise her/him what to buy.
3 Here is a list of six common causes of accidents to motorcyclists:
   a) drinking and riding
   b) going too fast for the traffic conditions
   c) making a mistake when turning or overtaking
   d) poor control of the machine (particularly on wet or icy roads)
   e) riding with a scratched or heavily tinted visor
   f) not being seen in time by other drivers.
   Draw a picture, diagram or cartoon to illustrate each one and write a caption for each.

4   At what age can you ride a motorcycle? How do you obtain a
    provisional licence? Is it worth doing a training course? Where
    can you take the test? What do you have to do for the two parts
    of the motorcycle driving test? Find out the answers to these
    questions and prepare a short talk on 'Learning to ride a
    motorcycle'.

Road accidents

If you are first on the scene at a road accident, what should you
do?

How to handle an accident

Stop and follow the steps listed below. Quick efficient
application of first aid can save lives.

What to do

1   Stop. It is an offence not to stop if you are involved in an
    accident. Switch on your hazard warning lights so that
    other drivers can see you.
2   Look around you, take in everything: for example,
    casualties may have been thrown clear of a car or bike,
    even over a hedge, and a child may have fallen under a
    seat.
3   Check that casualties are not in any more danger –
    remove danger first and only if this is *not* possible move
    the casualty from the danger.
4   Decide which casualty is the most seriously injured and
    treat him according to the priorities on page 64.
5   Send someone to call the emergency services, giving
    accurate details.
6   Immobilise any cars and warn other traffic of the danger.

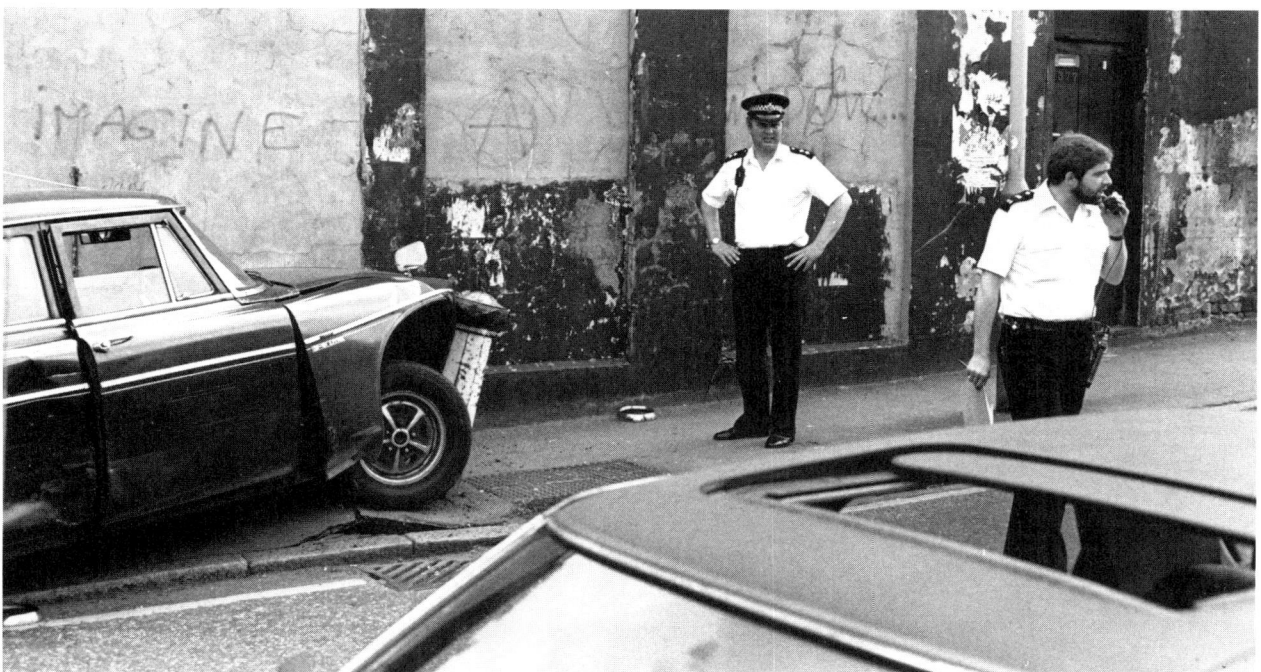

Know how to handle and help at a road accident.

Important

- Do not let anyone smoke near an accident; there may be petrol, oil or chemicals spilt on the road.
- Do not approach a casualty if it puts your life in danger.
- Do not move anything unless it is absolutely necessary. Make a note of the position before doing anything.

Priorities

The priorities for treating a casualty are listed below. However, in all incidents where there are several casualties you must treat the most seriously injured one first. Remember, the noisy casualty may not be the most seriously injured.

What to do

1   A.B.C. must be established immediately if the casuality is unconscious – permanent brain damage can occur after only three minutes without oxygen.
   a) The *Airway* (the passage between the mouth, nose, throat and windpipe) must be opened and kept open.
   b) *Breathing* must be established and maintained.
   c) *Circulation of blood* must be established and maintained. Severe bleeding must be stopped.
2   If the casualty needs to be moved, immobilise any broken bones before doing so.
3   Reassure the casualty and treat other injuries as required.

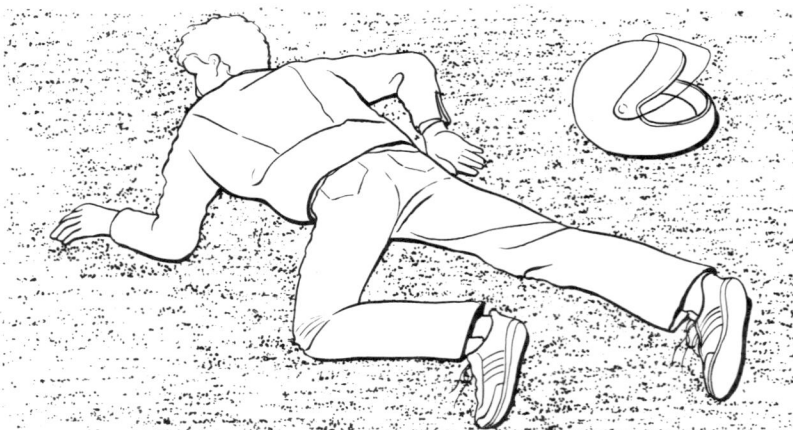

Points to look for

The following points will help you find out exactly what is wrong.

- History   How did the accident happen? Ask the casualty and any bystanders.
- Symptoms   Listen very carefully to everything the casualty tells you – is he in pain? Where is the pain? Can he move?
- Signs   Gently examine the casualty from head to foot, comparing one side of the body with the other. What can you see and feel? Look out for any medical warning signs such as a Medic-alert bracelet or S.O.S. Talisman.

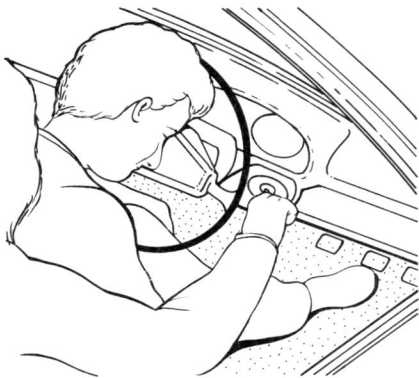

Further action

If you are first on the scene of an accident, not only is it important to give the casualty correct first aid as quickly as you can but also, as far as possible, to prevent fire breaking out and further collisions.

Minimise the risk of fire   Switch off the ignition; vehicles with diesel engines will have an emergency cut-off switch on the outside of the vehicle. Disconnect the battery because fires can start in the wiring. Gather together any fire extinguishers you find.

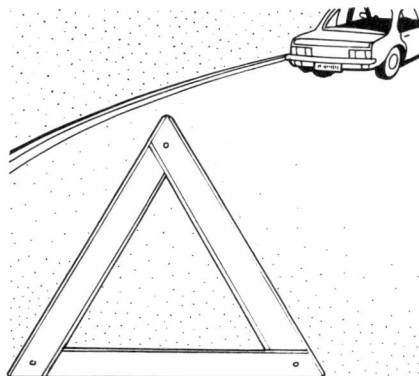

Warn other cars   Ask a bystander to set up a warning triangle at least 150 m (170 yd) back up the road from the accident. If there are no warning triangles, ask someone to direct traffic away from the accident.

Immobilise the car   Apply the handbrake and put the car into gear. Place blocks against the car wheels if there are any available. Do not try to right a car that has rolled on to its side.

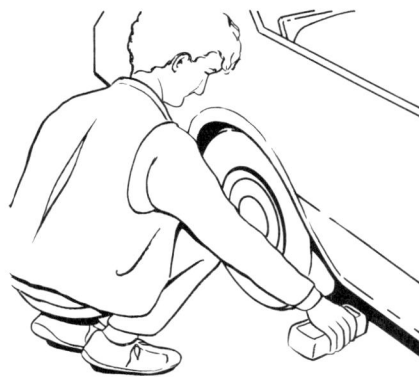

Witnesses   Get names and addresses of any witnesses so that they can be contacted later for statements. Do not leave this for too long after you have dealt with the casualty because people sometimes drift away.

Leaving the accident   Do not leave without obtaining permission from the police. If your vehicle is damaged, it must be checked for roadworthiness before driving away.

Tasks

1   Study the information on these pages.
   a) Prepare a short talk on how to deal with a road accident.
   b) Draw a flow chart showing what to do if you are first on the scene at an accident.
   c) Draw a picture-strip showing how a young person deals with a road accident in which two people are hurt.
2   How well do you know your Highway Code? Can you state
   a) two situations in which you should not overtake
   b) two things you should do when driving in fog
   c) two things you are not allowed to do on a motorway?
   Check your answers in a copy of the Highway Code. Then, make up your own ten question quiz and give it to a friend to do.

Safety at Work

Every employer has a duty to do everything possible to protect all employees. At the same time, employees must take reasonable care of their own safety and of everyone around.

Rights and responsibilities: The Health and Safety at Work Act 1974

The Act covers all people at work whether employers, workers or self-employed except for domestic servants in private households. It aims to protect not only people at work, but also the health and safety of the general public who may be affected by work activities. It lays down what are the general duties of employers, workers and manufacturers of equipment and chemicals.

Duties of employers

The main duty of an employer is to ensure as far as is reasonably practicable the health, safety and welfare at work of all her or his employees.

- The employer must provide workplaces, machines and methods of work that are safe and without risks to health. Any dangerous machinery must be properly guarded and all machines must be regularly serviced and maintained in good working order.
- The employer must make sure that machines and chemicals are used, stored and transported safely and without risks to health. For example, if the work involves a dangerous substance, such as asbestos, the employer must make sure that the safety procedures for working with asbestos are followed.
- The employer must provide a safe and healthy workplace with good welfare facilities. The workplace must have adequate heating, lighting and ventilation. The temperature must be reasonable to work in – neither too hot, nor too cold. The minimum temperature for workplaces is 16° C.
  The workplace must not be overcrowded. Welfare facilities such as toilets and washrooms should be provided, and the workplace must be kept clean.
- The employer must provide a workplace with safe entrances and exits. Fire precautions must be up to the approved standard, with fire alarms and extinguishers checked regularly and fire exits kept clear. Floors, stairs and gangways must be kept clear of obstructions. Clear instructions for the procedure in the event of a fire must be displayed and fire drills should be practised.
- Employees must be provided with the information, training and supervision necessary to ensure their health and safety. Your employer must make sure you know how to do your job, how to operate machines properly and make you aware of any potential dangers. You must know what the

accident procedures are and where the first aid box is kept.

- The employer must provide a written safety policy and make sure it is brought to the notice of all employees. Any person who employs five or more people has to prepare a written statement of her or his general policy, organisation and arrangements about health and safety at work. This must be revised and updated regularly.
- The employer must ensure that her or his firm's activities do not place the health or safety of any of the general public at risk. For example, any fumes or dust must be controlled. The disposal of waste products must be arranged so that they do not cause damage either to people or to the environment.

Case study – Peter

Peter was killed during his second day at work in a Birmingham factory. He was just seventeen. His chest was crushed when he got caught by a conveyor belt and dragged under a roller. He had received no training and no one was supervising him. There was no one to help him or switch off the machine when he got caught in it. No one to hear his cries for help.

The machine should have been guarded but the guard was missing. The management claim Peter must have removed it but the guard was on the other side of the machine and thick with dust. For a few extra pounds the machine could have had an automatic guard fitted that switched off the machine if the guard was moved or if someone was caught by the roller. The firm had decided it was too expensive.

Question

Do you think Peter was careless? Even if it was Peter who took off the guard, do you think he realised the danger? Which of the employer's duties towards their employees may the firm have failed to fulfil?

Duties of manufacturers

The manufacturers of machines, materials and chemicals must make sure that their products are safe.

- The product should be designed and manufactured properly so that it is safe and there are no risks to health.
- The product should be properly tested to make sure it is safe.
- Information should be supplied about the safety of the product and any precautions necessary for its safe use.

Task

Firms using vehicles to carry dangerous goods must display hazard information signs. Find out what these signs are and what they convey. (Use a copy of the Highway Code to check your answers.)

Duties of employees

The Health and Safety at Work Act lays down the duties of workers as well as of employers. As an employee it is your responsibility to do the following:

- To take reasonable care to avoid injury to yourself or your workmates.
- To follow the health and safety regulations that apply to your workplace.
- To co–operate with your employer to do everything possible to make the workplace safe.
- To behave in a sensible manner at all times and not to misuse anything that is provided to make your work safe.

If an accident happens because you did not follow the correct safety procedures, it is not just your employer who might be prosecuted. You might be prosecuted too.

Safety representatives

If there is a union at your workplace, the union can appoint or elect a safety representative. The safety representative has the following rights:

- To investigate potential hazards and dangerous incidents and to find out why an accident happens.
- To investigate complaints from any employee he or she represents about health and safety matters.
- To raise any matters about health and safety at the workplace with the employer.

Inspectors

The Act gives inspectors the right to enter any workplace which she or he thinks it necessary to enter in order to ensure that the Act is being observed. The inspector does not need to give any warning of a visit and does not need the owner's or occupier's permission to carry out an inspection.

If the workplace is unsafe for some reason, the inspector can do various things.

1   *A prohibition notice* is issued when the inspector discovers an activity that could lead to serious personal injury. The activity is prohibited until action has been taken to remove the danger. A prohibition notice can be served on the person involved in the activity or on the person in charge of the workplace at the time the notice is served.

2   *An improvement notice* is issued when an inspector discovers something wrong with either the equipment or the workplace that makes it unsafe. The inspector can state what must be done to put the matter right. The notice gives a deadline for the fault to be put right.

3 In addition to, or instead of, issuing a prohibition notice or an improvement notice the inspector can prosecute any person who is not observing the provisions of the Act.

4 The inspector can also seize, render harmless or destroy any article or materials considered so dangerous that they might cause personal injury at any moment.

PROHIBITION NOTICE

HEALTH AND SAFETY EXECUTIVE
Health and Safety at Work etc. Act 1974, Sections 22—24

Name and address (See Section 46)	To ..... C. J. Doe and Sons Ltd. .... Rooks Farm, Stapleup, Downshire ....
(a) Delete as necessary	(a) Trading as ... N/A ....
(b) Inspector's full name	I (b) ... John Everyman ....
(c) Inspector's official designation	one of (c) ... HM Agricultural Inspectors ....
(d) Official address	of (d) ...... Health & Safety Executive, Government Buildings, ... South Road, Lindon, Upshire ...... tel no. .... 06-567 4289 ....

hereby give you notice that I am of the opinion that the following activities,

namely:— .. use of a Sparkey MK II Battery Charger ....
.... Serial No 123456 ....
....
....

which are (a)~~being~~ ~~carried on~~ ~~by~~ ~~you~~/about to be carried on by you/~~under your control~~

(e) Location of activity	at (e) .... Rooks Farm, Stapleup, Downshire ....

~~involve~~, or will involve (a)~~being~~/an imminent risk, of serious personal injury.
I am further of the opinion that the said matters involve contraventions of the following statutory provisions:—

... Health & Safety at Work etc Act 1974 Section 2(1) ....
....
....

because .. on 10 November 1978 the battery charger was not ....
.... maintained adequately to ensure so far as is ....
.... reasonably practicable the safety of your employees ....

and I hereby direct that the said activities shall not be carried on by you or under your control (a) immediately/~~after~~

(f) Date	(f) ....

unless the said contraventions and matters included in the schedule, which forms part of this notice, have been remedied.

Signature ... J Everyman .... Date .... 11 November 1978 ..

LP 2	being an inspector appointed by an instrument in writing made pursuant to Section 19 of the said Act and entitled to issue this notice.

specimen prohibition notice

1   'It's not up to me. It's up to my employer to see that I'm safe at work and that safety regulations are observed.' Is this statement true or false? Explain why.
2   List the things a union safety representative is able to do in order to look after the health and safety of union members.
3   'No one can enter an employer's premises without permission.' Is this statement true or false? Explain why.
4   What is the difference between a prohibition notice and an improvement notice?
5   For what reasons can an inspector
    a) prosecute an employer
    b) destroy materials at a workplace?

Task

If you have an accident at work and your employer is found to be negligent you may be entitled to industrial injuries benefit or compensation. Find out what they are and how to obtain them.

Safety in the workshop

Each year over half a million people are injured in accidents at work. The following safety rules apply particularly to the operation and maintenance of machine tools such as lathes, milling machines and shaping machines.

Personal safety

Do

1   Immediately report *any* accidents, however small.
2   Wear safety glasses.
3   Wear safety footwear.
4   Use the barrier cream provided.
5   Wear your overalls buttoned up to protect your clothing and prevent loose clothing and ties becoming caught in moving parts of machines.
6   Either roll up your overall sleeves or button up the cuffs.
7   Keep your hair short or wear a cap, net or headband.

Do not

1   Do not wear rings or watches whilst operating a machine.
2   Do not keep sharp tools in your overall pockets.
3   Do not remove swarf with bare hands, use a brush.
4   Do not manually lift heavy equipment.
5   Do not lean on the machine.

Machine safety

Do

1   Keep machines and all equipment clean, and in good condition.
2   Before starting a machine ensure that you know how to stop it.
3   Switch off the machine immediately anything goes wrong.
4   Keep the machine and surrounding area tidy.
5   Check oil levels before first starting machines.

6 Switch off machines at mains at end of each day.
7 Check that chucks or cutters rotate in the correct direction before commencing cutting operations.
8 Use the correct tool or cutter for the job.
9 Replace tools that are worn or damaged.

Do not

1 Do not attempt to operate a machine until you know how to use it correctly.
2 Do not tamper with a machine.
3 Do not remove any stops in an effort to obtain a greater cutting range, or the machine may be seriously damaged.
4 Do not try and reverse the direction of a spindle while it is in motion.
5 Do not try to change a spindle speed while it is in motion.
6 Do not throw things.
7 Do not walk away and leave your machine running.
8 Do not direct compressed air at yourself or workmates. It can kill.

Tasks

1 Work with a partner. Study the safety rules. Suggest reasons for each one.
2 Where would you see these signs? State what each one means and in what kind of job or workplace the sign would be used.
3 Workers on building sites are more likely to be killed in accidents than workers in factories. Suggest why. What do you think are the main causes of accidents on building sites?
4 Make lists of potential safety hazards in each of the following workplaces:
   a) a canteen
   b) an office
   c) a shop
   d) a warehouse
   e) a factory
   f) a college or school
   g) a farm

2 a)

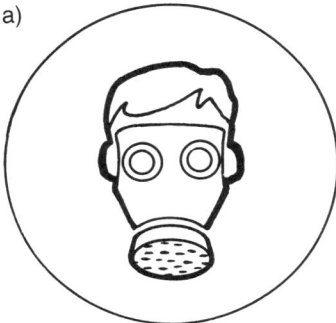

b)

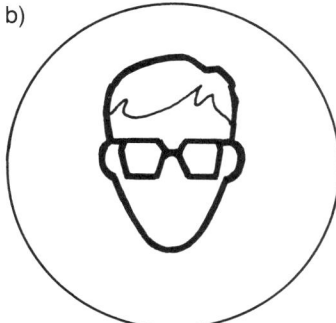

c)

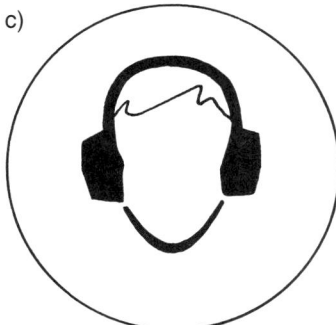

d)

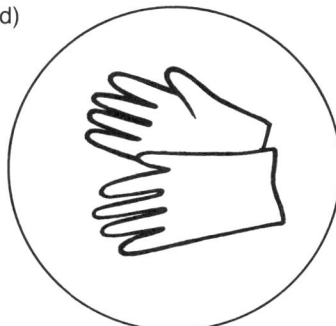

e)

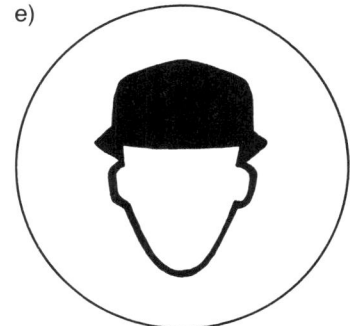

Back problems

About 70% of the population suffer back pain at some point during their working lives. It is estimated that over 15 million working days are lost each year through back strain.

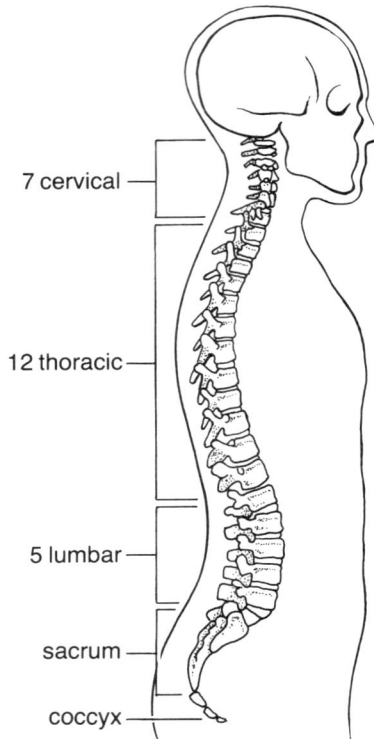

diagram of the spine

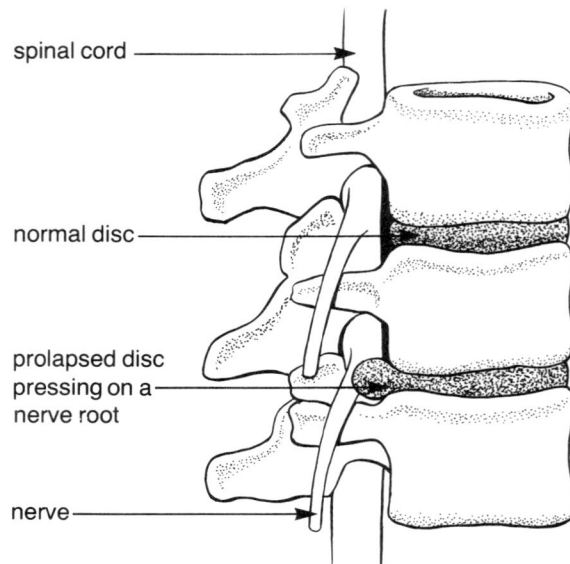

diagram showing a normal and prolapsed disc

Your back

The spine is an engineering miracle. It is made up of 24 movable vertebrae supporting the head at the top and resting on the pelvis below. The spine is arranged in three curves – one in the neck (*the cervical curve*), one in the chest (*the thoracic curve*), and one in the lumbar region. These curves help to absorb the stress put on the human spine because of man's erect posture. In addition, the spine is the basic framework of the body upon which everything else is anchored. It is also a flexible tunnel protecting the spinal cord and enabling nerves to be distributed to the rest of the body.

Discs

The discs act both as shock absorbers and spacers between the vertebrae.

Misuse of the spine

In a machine, if one small part functions wrongly, then the efficiency of the whole can be impaired. In the same way, if any structure around the spine is damaged, then the function of the whole is impaired. Damage and pain usually seem to be caused by sudden stress. But this stress may really be the last straw to an already insiduously damaged spine. If the spine is repeatedly misused, there is an accumulation of minor wear and tear, such as that caused by poor working position, bad posture or being overweight.

The most common cause of back injuries is lifting. If you lift something too heavy you may damage your spine by putting too much strain on it. If you lift something awkwardly or too quickly you may damage your spine by twisting or jerking it.

Rules for lifting

1 Before you lift a load, remove any obstacles that may be in the way.
2 Always keep a straight back when lifting, pushing or pulling. Bend your knees, not your back.
3 When you are lifting, keep the load as close to your body as possible.
4 The best height for a load to be lifted is 40 cm above ground level. All loads should be rested on a convenient platform from which they can be picked up again.
5 If any hoists or mechanical aids are available, always use them rather than brute strength.
6 Never attempt to lift anything which is too heavy for you.

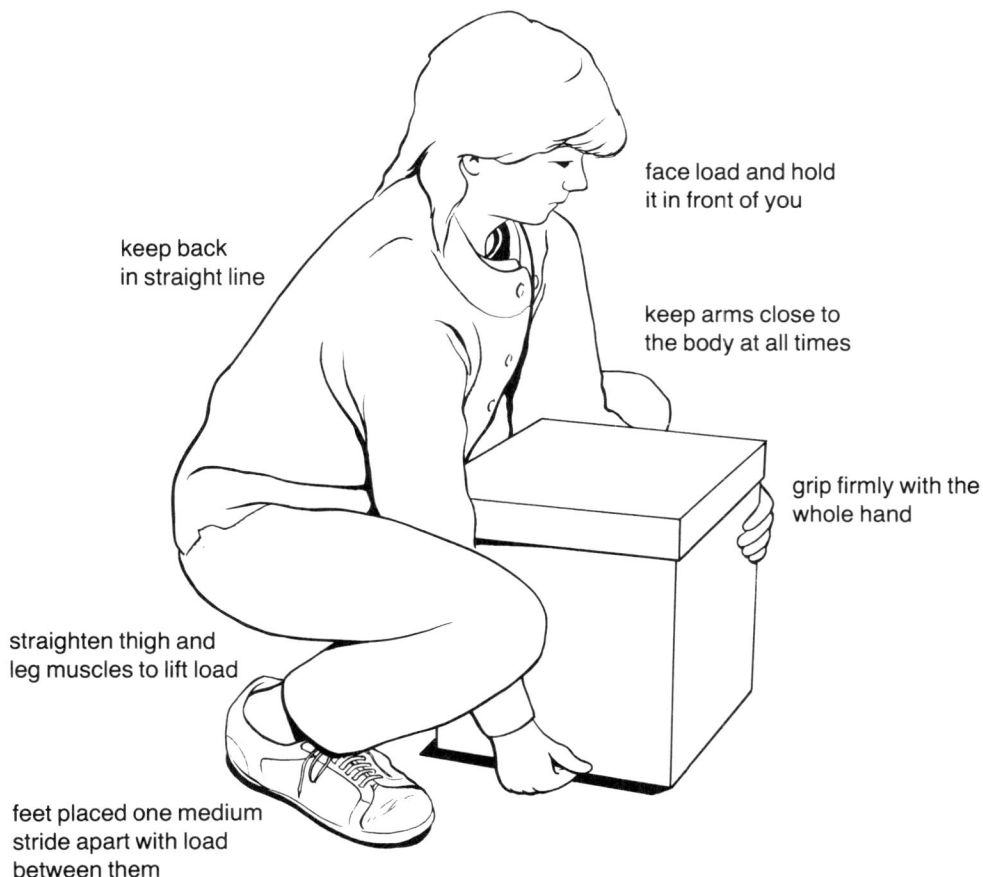

keep back in straight line

face load and hold it in front of you

keep arms close to the body at all times

grip firmly with the whole hand

straighten thigh and leg muscles to lift load

feet placed one medium stride apart with load between them

correct lifting position

Working surfaces

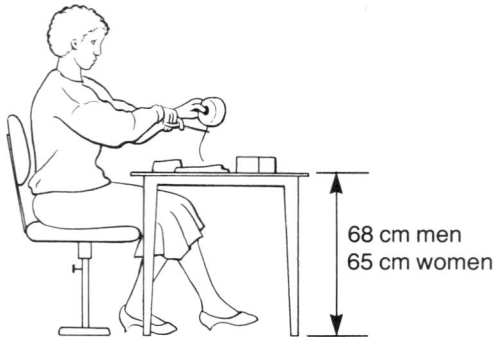

This shows the right height for a work surface for manual work. The measurements are for men and women of average height.

68 cm men
65 cm women

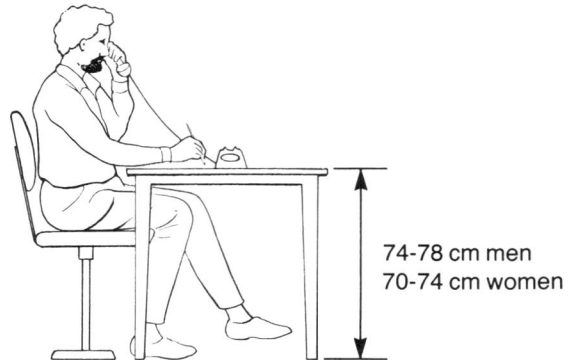

This is the recommended height for drawing, reading, writing and eating.

74-78 cm men
70-74 cm women

delicate work

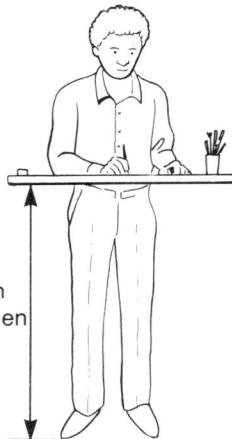

100-110 cm men
95-105 cm women

light manual

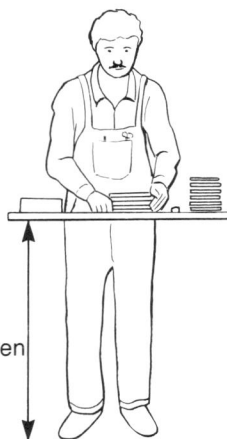

90-95 cm men
85-90 cm women

heavy manual

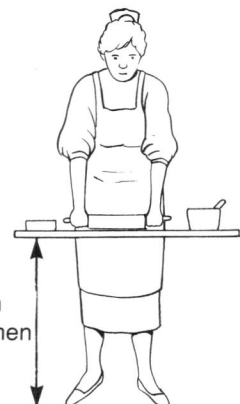

75-90 cm men
70-85 cm women

These are the right heights for standing at work.

Tasks

1 Study the rules for lifting. Suggest reasons for each one.
2 a) Carry out a survey to find out if it appears to be true that 70% of the working population suffer back pain at some time in their working lives. Try to find out how each person injured her or his back, how serious the injury was, what treatment each person has had to have and how the injury has affected her or his life.
   b) Does your survey suggest that people in certain jobs are more at risk than others? List the jobs in which back injuries appear more likely to occur.
3 Measure the height of a number of different tables and workbenches in rooms in your college or school. In which room(s) are the working surfaces at the most suitable and least suitable heights?
4 If a work surface is at the wrong height for you, what can you do?

Safety at work – Noise

It is estimated that about 30 million workers in the EEC are exposed to undesirable noise levels and about 10 million to noise levels which damage their hearing.

How is noise measured?

Noise is measured in units called *decibels*. In the decibel scale, each ten decibels multiples the level of noise by ten. So a noise of 90 decibels is ten times louder than a noise of 80 decibels and 1000 times louder than a noise of 60 decibels.

How dangerous is noise?

A person who works for eight hours a day at a noise level of 110 decibels for ten years will probably lose 50% of her or his hearing ability. A government code of practice for reducing the exposure of workers to noise lays down 90 decibels as the average level of noise to which a worker should be exposed during an eight hour day. But exposure even at this level is likely to cause damage to hearing over a number of years.

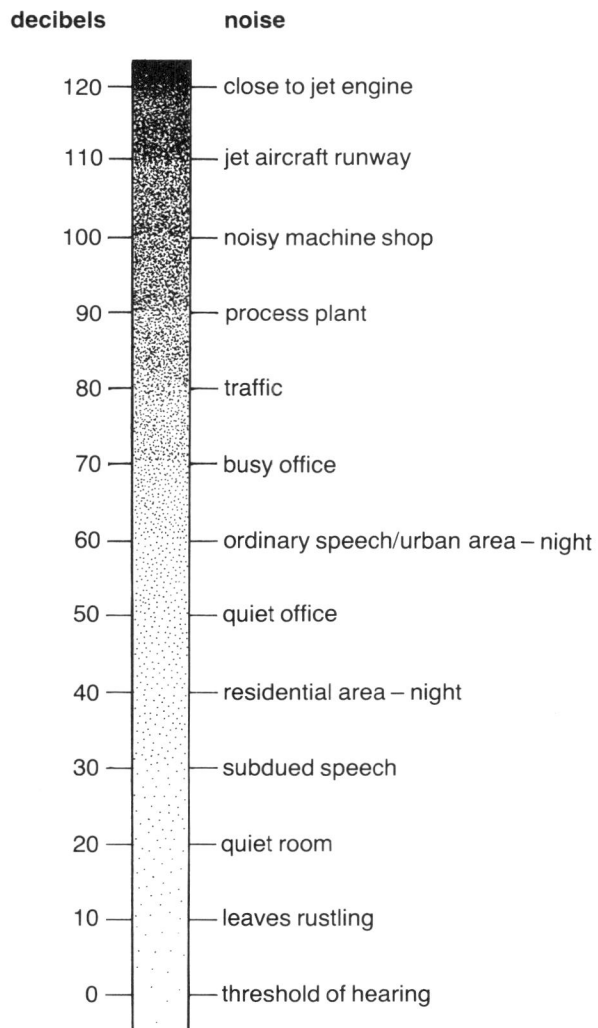

decibels	noise
120	close to jet engine
110	jet aircraft runway
100	noisy machine shop
90	process plant
80	traffic
70	busy office
60	ordinary speech/urban area – night
50	quiet office
40	residential area – night
30	subdued speech
20	quiet room
10	leaves rustling
0	threshold of hearing

How can noise be controlled?

As well as damaging hearing, noise causes stress. The solution to the problem of noise is to remove the hazard by soundproofing and by improving the design of machinery and of workplaces.

If you work in noisy conditions, wear the ear protectors which are provided. But ear protectors are only a short-term solution to the problem of noise. It is impossible to wear them for long periods and at high noise levels they are of only limited use.

Questions

1   If you are going to a disco or a rock concert, do you ever wear ear plugs?
    What are the arguments for and against wearing them?
2   If you are worried about noise levels at work, what should you do?
3   If you are worried by noise from your neighbours or from a nearby construction site, what should you do?

Illness at work – Stress

Every year up to 5 million working days are lost due to illnesses which are related to stress.

What is stress?

At its simplest stress is similar to being excited. Your body releases *adrenalin*, a hormone, and this causes your heart rate to increase and blood to be diverted away from your stomach and face into the brain, and arm and leg muscles. Your muscles tense, you breathe a bit more quickly and you go pale. This reaction is called your 'fight or flight' mechanism.

You get a shock and your body immediately gets ready for action. Blood to the brain to speed thinking, to the arms and legs to get ready to run or fight. However, if the stress goes on for long periods or happens regularly this reaction can lead to other symptoms.

Being continually 'ready for action' tires you out and a simple short-term effect of stress is to make you feel exhausted even if you haven't done much exercise. The tension may give you a headache, stiff muscles or a backache. Because the blood is diverted away from your stomach you may get indigestion. The longer and more often you face stress the worse these problems may become.

Headaches may become migraines. Indigestion may become ulcers. You may develop high blood pressure and become more prone to heart attacks. Some people suffer nervous rashes or asthma. Some develop facial twitches. Extreme stress can also cause nervous breakdowns and anxiety neurosis.

What causes stress at work?

The main causes of stress at work are the conditions of work, the speed of work, how boring or demanding the work is and the effect of your job on your family and social life.

Some causes of stress	Some effects
• Overwork, long hours, poor diet • Pace of work too fast • Too much responsibility, over-promotion • Unsatisfying, monotonous, boring or meaningless work • Isolation from workmates, lack of release from tension in talk or organising • Lack of control over pace of production and conditions of work • Insecurity and anxiety about job, redundancies, takeovers, retraining, money, retirement, pension • Environment-noise, vibrations, heat, cold, poor lighting • Narcotic and other chemicals affecting nervous system • Fear of hazards, disease and injury • Domestic problems resulting from shiftwork or excessive overtime	• Fatigue • Accidents • Ulcers • Indigestion • High blood pressure • Heart attack • Skin rash • Backache • Depression • Anxiety neurosis • Headaches • Migraine • Asthma

Water Safety

It is important to remember that there are possible dangers connected with water, whether it is swimming, fishing, boating or just walking on a river bank. Watch out for the danger and learn what to do in an emergency for your own safety and the safety of others.

At home

It is possible for a baby or a toddler to drown in only a few inches of water. Young children should never be left alone in the bathroom. If the phone rings or there is a knock at the door, take the child out of the bath before going to see who it is.

Tragedies can easily happen in garden ponds, water troughs or paddling pools. To guard against accidents, ponds should either be fenced off or covered with strong wire mesh. Paddling pools should be kept empty when not in use and children should never be left unattended when playing in a paddling pool. Deep holes and disused wells should be securely covered.

Water sports

Sporting accidents may be caused by ignorance, irresponsible behaviour and neglecting to observe the basic rules of safety. Make sure you are aware of the possible dangers on or beside the water.

Swimming safety

- Always go swimming with someone else. Never go swimming alone.
- Do not go swimming if you are feeling tired or ill.
- Do not stay in the water too long. Get out as soon as you start to feel cold.
- Keep away from areas where there are boats, windsurfers or people fishing.
- Do not go swimming in disused gravel pits or quarries.
- Do not take any air-beds or inflatables into the sea.
- Before swimming at the seaside, ask about the tides and currents.
- Never ignore any warning signals or danger signs.
- Always swim in line with the shore.
- Do not go for a swim until at least an hour after a meal.
- Do not dive straight in at places where you haven't been swimming before.
- Never do things just to try to impress people.
- Never throw another person into the water. Accidents can occur if the water is too shallow. The results can be concussion, broken bones or at least bruising and shock.

Boating safety

Boating accidents may be caused by ignorance and inability to handle the craft, lack of proper life-saving equipment, people behaving irresponsibly or foolishly and unsafe craft.

- Before you set out make sure everybody is wearing sensible clothes. Everyone should have warm and waterproof clothing and should wear a life-jacket which conforms to British Standards.
- The person in charge must know how to manage the boat properly and know the local conditions such as the tides and currents, the coastline and any local hazards, where the coastguards are and what the weather forecast is.
- The boat and all its equipment, including lifebelts, fire extinguishers, lights, signals, repair kit, first aid kit and navigating equipment (maps, charts) must be in good working order.
- You should tell somebody where you are going and what time you intend to return.
- Everyone on the boat should know what the emergency drill is and what to do if there is an accident.

Water rescue

- If you fall in the water or get into trouble in the water keep calm. If you panic, you increase the chances that you will drown before someone can help you. You should lie on your back and float. Then, try to attract attention by shouting for help and waving with one of your arms.

- If someone else falls into the water or gets into trouble in the water, do not immediately jump into the water to try to help. Many of the people who drown each year do so because they jump in to try to rescue other people who are in difficulties.

  A lot of drowning accidents happen within five metres of safety. If the person is close enough to the bank or shore, look round to see if there is an object you could use to reach her or him – perhaps a paddle, a stick or a scarf. If there is, lie down on the bank so that you won't be pulled in yourself and use it to pull the person to safety.

  If the person is too far out, try to throw her or him something to cling onto such as a lifebelt. Then, summon emergency help from either the police or the coastguard service.

- If you get someone to safety and find that breathing has stopped give mouth-to-mouth resuscitation immediately. If there is no heart beat, give heart massage. If the person is unconscious but still breathing, put her or him in the recovery position (see page 64) and wait for help to arrive.

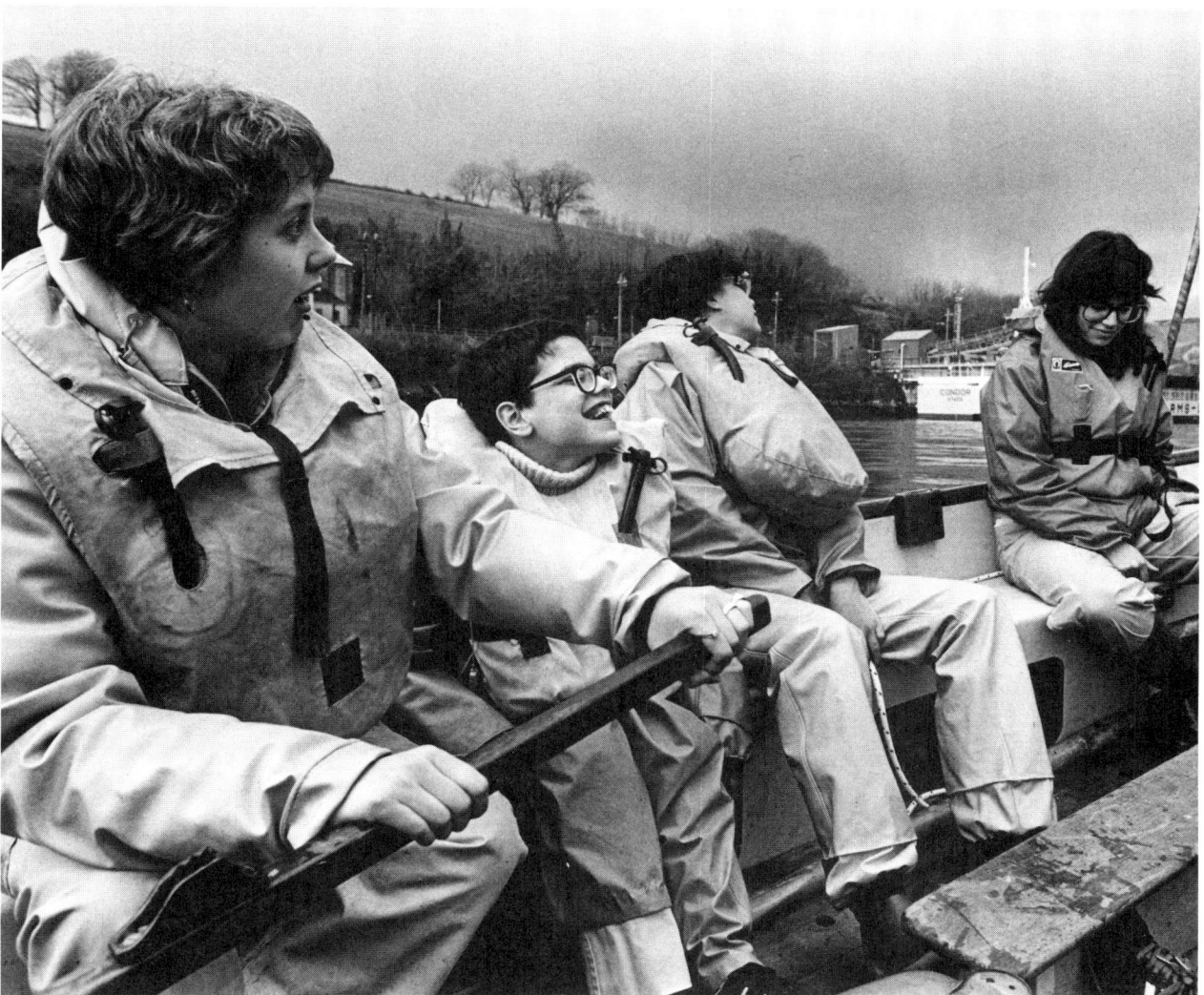

You need to wear the proper safety clothing when boating.

Questions

1 Study the advice on swimming safety. Work out the reasons for each piece of advice.

2 State what you would do in each of these situations:
a) You are lying on the beach. You see someone on an air-bed drifting out to sea.
b) You are out for a walk. You see someone sliding on a frozen pond fall through the ice.
c) You are fishing on a river bank. You hear a cry and realise that someone has fallen into the river.
d) You are swimming in a lake. You have gone further out than you thought and are having difficulty getting back within your depth.
e) You are out on a boat when you are hit by a wave which causes it to capsize.

3 A friend is planning to hire a boat to take out on the sea for a day. List all the things that should be checked before setting out.

Tasks

1 Find a first aid manual. Look up how to do mouth-to-mouth resuscitation. For how long should you do mouth-to-mouth resuscitation?

2 If you want to take up a water-sport such as windsurfing, sailing or canoeing, you are advised to join a club. Why? Find out about the opportunities there are for water sports in your area.